Praise for Pain Free Formula

"The Pain-Free Formula bridges the critical gaps often overlooked in traditional pain management. Stacey Roberts expertly connects new evidence-based elements, providing practical solutions and insights that are both accessible and transformative. As a physical therapist specializing in orthopedics and sports medicine, I value how this book empowers readers with the tools to understand and address pain. It's an essential guide for anyone committed to staying or becoming active again for long-term well-being and happiness."
—Kim MacDonald MPT, DPT

"As a pharmacist and wellness coach, I found *The Pain-Free Formula* to be an invaluable resource for anyone grappling with pain. Stacey Roberts masterfully makes complex concepts easy to understand and tackles valuable information about pharmaceuticals and surgeries that are not often discussed. This clarity empowers readers to make informed choices in their care. Importantly, Stacey does not discount the value of medical expertise; instead, she complements it by offering additional information and solutions that enhance overall outcomes. This is a wonderful resource not only for anyone experiencing pain but also for any provider helping their patients. I wholeheartedly recommend The *Pain Free Formula* as a must-read for those looking to transform their relationship with pain and pursue a healthier future."
—Gina Lynn Lusis, RPh, Holistic Health Coach

"I deeply appreciate how *The Pain-Free Formula* connects the mind and body in addressing pain. As a mental health therapist, I find the author's focus on new research and powerful tools to help those suffering from pain truly inspiring. This book is an invaluable resource for anyone seeking to heal on a deeper level."
—Chelsey Roberts LPC, MS, MSc

"Stacey Roberts is a trusted colleague whose work I deeply admire. In *The Pain Free Formula*, she masterfully breaks down the intricate relationship between hormones and pain, offering insightful and compassionate guidance to those who need it most. Stacey's vast experience, combined with her holistic approach, makes this book an essential resource for anyone struggling with chronic pain. Her innovative techniques and genuine care have the power to create lasting transformation. If you're ready to reclaim your health and discover lasting relief, this is the book you've been waiting for."

—Patty Aubery, CEO of The Canfield Training Group
and co-author of Permission Granted

The Pain Free Formula

The
Pain Free
Formula

Solving the Puzzle of Muscle and Joint Pain
Without Surgery, Drugs or Injections

Stacey Roberts PT, RN, MSN

Medical Disclaimer:
This book is for general informational purposes only and does not constitute the practice of medicine, nursing, or other professional health care services, including the giving of medical advice. No provider-patient relationship is formed with the use of this information, and the materials linked to this book are at the user's own risk. The content in this book is not intended to be a substitute for professional medical advice. Readers should not disregard or delay in obtaining medical advice related to any medical condition they have, and they should seek the assistance of their healthcare professionals for any such conditions. Names and identifying characteristics of individuals throughout this book have been changed to protect their privacy.

Copyright © 2025 by Stacey Roberts PT, RN, MSN

All rights reserved. No part of this book may be used or reproduced by any means, graphic, electronic, or mechanical, including photocopying, recording, taping, or by any information storage retrieval system, without the written permission of the copyright holder, except in the cases of brief quotations embodied in critical articles and reviews. No version of this book (including the audio version) may be used for training AI.

Published by Positive Image Publishing
6650 W State St Suite 233
Wauwatosa, WI 53213

ISBN (paperback): 978-0-9981837-1-8
ISBN (ebook): 978-0-9981837-2-5

Book design and production by www.AuthorSuccess.com

Printed in the United States of America

This book is dedicated to my patients, family, friends, co-workers, Joe Tate, my business partner, and my son. You all continue to inspire me to be the best I can be. Thank you!

For more information and a FREE discovery call go to www.newyouhealthandwellness.com
Email: Info@newyouhealthandwellness.com
414-299-8121

Contents

Foreword	*xiii*
Introduction	*1*

PART ONE: Exposing the Current Pain Paradigm — 9

Chapter 1:	Unmasking Your Pain	13
Chapter 2:	Wired For Warning: How Pain Works	20
Chapter 3:	What Your Doctor May Not Have Told You About the Conventional Treatment of Your Pain	33
Chapter 4:	Surgical Shadows	74

PART TWO: The New Pain Paradigm — 95

Chapter 5:	Why Won't My Pain Go Away?	102
Chapter 6:	Biomechanics and Insufficient Movement Patterns	118
Chapter 7:	SoftWave: The Most Effective Modality to Get Rid of Localized Pain	128
Chapter 8:	Tackling the Intangible Triggers	172
Chapter 9:	Gut Health and Joint/Muscle Pain	185
Chapter 10:	When Good Food is Bad for You	213
Chapter 11:	How Hormones Cause Joint and Muscle Pain	232
Chapter 12:	When Stress Takes a Toll	274
Chapter 13:	The Brain and Your Pain	297

Afterword	339
Sources	342

Foreword

By Molly Fay, host of *The Morning Blend* on WTMJ-TV, Milwaukee's NBC Affiliate

I first met Stacey Roberts in my role as co-host of *The Morning Blend*. She came on our show to discuss pelvic and sexual health—an important topic, though not one I personally needed at the time. What struck me, even then, was Stacey's deep commitment to helping people and her passion for addressing issues others often shy away from.

But the next time Stacey appeared on the show, I paid much closer attention. This time, she was talking about her unique program that reduced inflammation and relieved pain. It was the kind of conversation that made me sit up and take notice, because I'd been struggling with ankle pain and swelling for over a decade. Ten years of treatments, MRIs, and frustration, yet nothing seemed to help. Could Stacey's system *really* make a difference for me? I wasn't convinced. But something about Stacey—her knowledge, her confidence, and her genuine care—gave me hope.

I made the call. What did I have to lose? A little time, a little money. But maybe, just maybe, I could gain something back: the ability to walk pain-free, to live without constant swelling, and to reclaim my favorite activities.

You can read the full details of my journey with Stacey in Chapter 7, but I'll give you this much: Stacey changed my life. Her treatments, combined with her thoughtful, integrative approach, took my pain from debilitating to nearly nonexistent. My once-swollen ankle, which looked more like an elephant's foot rather than my own, finally started to heal *after ten years* of struggling. And I wasn't just walking again—I was walking *five miles*, pain-free, through the beautiful streets of Charleston on an anniversary trip with my husband.

What makes Stacey—and this book—so unique is her evidence-based, deeply experienced approach. She treats the site of chronic pain AND she uncovers its true root cause while crafting a personalized program to resolve it.

The *Pain-Free Formula* offers an incredible understanding of the body as a whole—how hormones drive inflammation and impact joint health, how gut imbalances contribute to chronic pain, and how we can support the body's natural ability to heal. It also reveals how pharmaceutical drugs and surgeries, while sometimes necessary, can fail to address the root causes of pain. But more importantly, this book delivers real, actionable solutions to help you find lasting relief.

This isn't a quick-fix book about masking pain. Stacey truly listens to her patients, as evidenced not only by my personal experience with her, but also the conversations she reveals in *The Pain-Free Formula*. She empowers you to uncover what's happening *beneath the surface by placing the often-overlooked pieces of the pain puzzle in the right place to move you to where you want to be*. She educates readers about inflammation, the role of hormones, gut health, stress, and the impact of lifestyle choices so that healing becomes both possible and sustainable.

For me, Stacey's program was nothing short of a game-changer. I'm walking, practicing yoga, and moving through life with far less pain. And on many days . . . pain-free. If you're ready to reclaim your health and finally find lasting relief, *The Pain-Free Formula*, filled with real-life stories, practical knowledge, and expert tips, introduces you to a revelatory daily practice and shows you how to make it work for your modern life.

Molly Fay
The Morning Blend

Introduction

Did you ever stumble upon a moment that seemed like an unwelcome event, only to realize it was the key to reshaping your perspective?

On July 31, 2021, I was at a lively and beautiful barn wedding reception for my niece and her long-time beau. The music was a blend of fun country music and Midwest classics. My son was in his twenties and having a ball with his cousins on the dance floor. Although new to a Wisconsin wedding tradition, the polka, he was more than willing to give it his best shot, as multiple Brandy Manhattans decreased any fear of embarrassment he might have otherwise felt. As I watched him struggle to find his footing, I decided to jump out of my seat and show him the ropes. After a minute or two of the one-two-two, one-two-two rhythm while we were smiling, sweating, and laughing on the barnyard wooden floor, I suddenly felt a 'pop,' accompanied by a searing pain piercing through my knee. Since my one-two-two rhythm abruptly stopped, my son, having sensed the change in my cadence, leaned in toward my ear and yelled above the music, "Are you okay?"

Holding desperately onto his hands to stay upright, I leaned in and yelled, "I just felt a huge pop in my knee."

His eyes widened, as he wasn't used to seeing my face crinkle in pain. Silently, he started to help me off the dance floor, but I shooed him away to go have fun with his friends.

As I limped to a nearby table, hoping I could walk it off, each step felt like a nail was driving its way through the inside of my knee. As I approached the white, cloth-covered table, I realized this was significantly worse than I had thought. Grabbing a metal folding chair, it screeched across the floor as I pulled it toward me. I slowly lowered myself onto it, and my royal blue dress hiked up naturally. My eyes fell to my right knee as it was fast becoming twice the size of my left. My experience as a physical therapist kicked in and I knew I needed to get back to my hotel to ice and elevate it. The throbbing persisted, and as I thought about getting up, tears welled up, my throat tightened, and I closed my eyes, asking for strength and praying for the pain to subside. I took a deep breath, and as I stood up, I became a bit dizzy and nauseous from what now felt like a shard of glass shoved into my joint.

After a few seconds, while standing, I took another deep breath, let it out, and with a strained smile excused myself, determined to reach my car and call it a night.

Once out of the barn, I kicked off my small, wedged heels and they clicked and clacked while bouncing down the staircase. Then, I proceeded to hop down each step on my left leg and retrieved my shoes at the bottom. Dragging my leg behind me as I walked toward the parking lot, I was trying to think of anything but the jabbing feeling in my knee. I halted and caught my breath. As I looked ahead to my car many yards away, I stood only bearing weight on my left leg like some sort of six-foot-tall royal blue flamingo. Humor, another tactic to distract me from what now felt like a fifty-pound weight around my right lower extremity, worked a bit, and honestly, I am not sure how, but I made it to my car.

After getting in, I was forced to awkwardly manipulate the brake and gas pedals with my left foot as I navigated my way back to the motel. My arrival was no respite; every step was agony so a lot of hopping ensued. Thankfully, the foyer was empty, and I found every piece of furniture I could to assist me while making my way toward and into the elevator.

As I traveled up to my floor, I felt my chest heaving and sweat dripping down my sides and my back. *At least I was burning some calories*, I thought.

With the ding of the elevator door opening, I hopped to the vending area and filled an empty Walgreens plastic bag I took from my car with ice. Outside my hotel room, I fumbled for my key, laid it flat against the sensor, and pushed the door open so I could bounce to my bed. As I hoisted my leg up onto two pillows to elevate it, I placed the leaking bag of ice on my ballooning knee. Water started trickling out in tiny streams around my leg, and the cool sensation seemed to travel through all the blood vessels in my body. I did not mind the intense burning I felt from the ice, as the tissue it covered began to go numb. After it was wrapped tight against the injured area, I fell back onto my pillows.

Ladies and gentlemen . . . the Beer Barrel Polka took me out.

A restless night followed, prompting my son to take a trip to pick up the crutches I had ordered online. My bloated knee refused to allow my limb to bear weight, and the journey home was a symphony of melting ice and searing discomfort. Desperate, I traveled to my clinic, where I turned to my SoftWave machine, an electrohydraulic shockwave device I had employed to the benefit of countless patients. I had hoped it could heal me, too. To my astonishment, as I stood after the first treatment, video footage will confirm that I heard myself mumble, "Huh." The pain had diminished while standing to a mere fraction of what it had been only thirty minutes before.

The throbbing and stabbing subsided gradually with each treatment. The progress was undeniable.

After a third session, I was able to walk without crutches. The pain, once roaring for my attention, had subsided to a mere whisper as I walked. My knee, though not entirely stable, was on the mend.

But uncertainty still lingered. As a seasoned physical therapist (PT) with over three decades of experience and a registered nurse, I wanted a thorough assessment. *What was that pop?* I wondered. So, I sought out an orthopedic surgeon, eager to find answers and discuss my situation with a fellow orthopedic expert. I was not going to let this injury turn into the type of chronic pain my patients, family members, and I had experienced before.

That pivotal moment and the unbelievably frustrating meeting I had with the orthopedic surgeon that followed marked the beginning of a journey that has led to a heightened personal commitment to my patients. This book is a large part of that commitment. Here, I accumulate thirty-plus years of knowledge and experience into unique solutions for chronic joint and muscle pain that I am sure your doctor hasn't talked to you about.

What to Expect Ahead

If you've ever been trapped in the cycle of suffering, tried surgeries, injections, and medication, *or* to avoid them, this book is for you.

The Pain-Free Formula: Solving the Puzzle of Muscle and Joint Pain without Surgery, Drugs, or Injections is not a tale of feeble promises, but a transformative educational journey rooted in real experiences, cutting-edge research, and expert knowledge.

You're about to unravel the mysteries associated with joint and muscle pain and embark on a path of relief that *you* have control over. Through my dual roles as a seasoned physical therapist and a master's prepared nurse, as well as having experienced and resolved bouts of significant muscle and joint pain myself, I've honed a revolutionary formula that combines emerging research, straightforward steps, and frankly, common sense, which does not always equate with medical sense, empowering you to reclaim a life free from the grip of pain.

Who am I? And why the heck should you listen to me?

My journey from pain to relief for myself and my patients allows me to have a unique perspective—one that seamlessly bridges the chasm between medical knowledge and personal understanding. As a lifelong athlete, I, too, have navigated chronic muscle and joint pain, confronting the same choices you face now, as have my patients over three decades. The weight of the medical establishment's verdict—surgery, drugs, injections—loomed over me and the patients I see daily as I searched for an alternative path.

I've witnessed firsthand that at times, pain can resist most conventional means of addressing it, but with some creativity and knowledge, it can often be relieved. The following pages are not just an aggregation of information, but a testament to an unwavering dedication to easing suffering and promoting well-being. As I've guided countless patients through their journeys, I hope *The Pain-Free Formula* will also help guide you successfully through yours.

What Will You Learn?

The Pain-Free Formula is a compass that shows you ways out of the maze of pain. The book is divided into two parts, each designed to unravel the intricate puzzle that pain presents and offer actionable solutions.

Part I, "Exposing the Current Pain Paradigm: Unveiling Current Conventional Approaches to Chronic Pain and Why It Doesn't Work for Many," dismantles myths, examines the reality of inflammatory muscle and joint conditions, and helps you understand why you still have pain. This section empowers you with knowledge, equipping you to confront the root cause of pain head-on with your team of healthcare providers.

As you transition to Part II, "The New Pain Paradigm: A Blueprint to Lasting Relief," you'll encounter a guide designed to liberate you from pain's grasp. From personalized strategies to cutting-edge modalities, and unique but extremely effective testing and evidence-based interventions that have helped me and countless others achieve relief, Part II is a testament to the profound shift in perspective that awaits you. With every chapter, you'll inch closer to finding the relevant pieces of your pain puzzle so you can find your path to the solutions you seek.

What's in It for You?

The Pain-Free Formula is not just a book; it's your roadmap to regaining a life untainted by suffering. By the end of the journey, you'll achieve the following:

- **Unlock the Mystery of Why You Still Have Pain**
  Understand the true origins of your pain. Discover the real reasons why you have it and haven't gotten rid of it while debunking misconceptions that have hindered your progress along the way.

- **Harness Holistic Healing**
  Begin to understand outside-of-the-box thinking supported by cutting-edge research you can apply to your everyday life that has been proven to lessen and eliminate chronic joint and muscle pain.

- **Evade the Surgical Abyss**
  Potentially escape surgery and invasive injections, discovering an alternative path toward healing.

- **Break Free from Medication**
  Liberate yourself, if possible, from long-term pain and anti-inflammatory medications that can have negative impacts on your health and, counterintuitively, make you *more* sensitive to

feeling pain. In their place, you will discover healthy alternatives to achieve your health goals.

- **Understand How to Address Pain Holistically**
  Discover how countless others have successfully addressed pain by following programs designed to find the true root cause of why you still have pain and what you can do about it.

- **Rediscover the Joy of an Active Life Again**
  The goal of this book is to help you become a full participant in your life again. By addressing and removing all the pain-provoking triggers discussed in these pages, you can get back to living the life you love.

As you immerse yourself in *The Pain-Free Formula*, remember that this is your journey towards a life where pain doesn't take center stage. The story I share is not just mine; it's one we all share, united by the yearning for an active and satisfying life beyond joint and muscle pain. I hope these pages will be your guide, inspiration, and beacon of hope. Your future, free from joint and muscle pain awaits.

AUTHOR'S NOTE:

Key Puzzle Pieces for Lasting Change

At the end of each chapter, you will see this puzzle piece symbol:

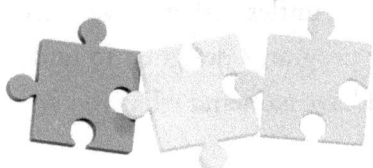

This indicates 'Key Pieces of the Puzzle'—a summary of the most important insights from that chapter. These key points are designed to reinforce essential concepts, providing you with a clearer understanding of the main takeaways and how they fit into the bigger picture of helping you create a Pain-Free life.

DISCLAIMER: Names have been changed to protect privacy, and none of the information in this book replaces an appointment with your healthcare provider, but I hope the educational details in these pages lead you to the answers you seek.

PART ONE
Exposing the Current Pain Paradigm

UNVEILING CURRENT CONVENTIONAL APPROACHES TO CHRONIC PAIN AND WHY IT DOESN'T WORK FOR MANY

> "When you change the way you look at things, the things you look at change."
>
> *Wayne Dyer*

At eighty-three years old, my mother lay breathless on her side, silently weeping due to what I imagined was a mix of embarrassment and frustration, doing her best to hide her experience that her once-strong body was now a battleground of pain. As I carefully lifted each of her swollen legs onto her bed, I felt a deep ache in my own heart—a pain that no medicine could soothe. Her knees, worn from years of tireless work around our home; her back, aching from decades as a nurse; and her shoulders, now fragile from severe arthritis, all bore the marks of a lifetime spent caring for others.

Every day, I witness pain—patients who have filled my schedule at the hospitals, sports clinics, and outpatient centers over the years. But nothing prepared me for the heartache of seeing my mother suffer. The woman who raised me, whose hands once held me steady, now needed mine to ease her back into bed. It felt as though someone was squeezing my heart, slowly tightening the vice until all I could do was pray for some relief for her.

We all age, and we all encounter pain to varying degrees. It's a part of life. But with today's advanced research and understanding, we have more opportunities than ever to address the root causes of the pain that regularly interferes with our lives, to seek relief not solely through a pill or an injection, but through the incredible healing power within our own bodies. When conventional methods fall short, there's a world of possibilities waiting to be explored; a world where answers are within reach.

Though my mother may believe it's too late, I refuse to give up on her—or on you. There is hope, there is healing, and there is a path to a life free from the burden of muscle and joint pain. This book is my promise to you, a guide to finding relief, and a testament to the belief that there is a light ahead, just right around the corner.

Welcome to *The Pain-Free Formula*. If you picked up this book, it's likely because you are searching for answers, for relief, or for hope. And I am here to tell you—you are not alone, and there is a way forward.

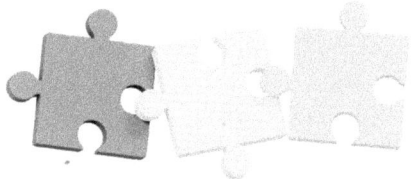

Key Pieces

Pain stinks. And in a healthcare world that has a tendency to focus mostly on treating symptoms and not the underlying cause of your pain, you may feel like you've tried everything: countless doctors, myriad treatments, and various remedies, all without relief.

This book aims to change that.

In Part One of *The Pain-Free Formula*, you will find new answers to some of the most frustrating questions that patients dealing with muscle and joint pain have, and in Part Two, you'll learn the four areas that must be assessed and addressed to finally get rid of the pain. So, let's get started.

CHAPTER 1
Unmasking Your Pain

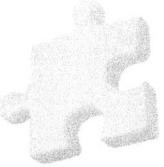

"Although the world is full of suffering, it is also full of the overcoming of it."

–Helen Keller

When Jean limped into my clinic, her story unfolded like many others, yet like all my patients, it remained uniquely her own. The latter part of midlife had brought not only wisdom but a longing to reconnect with the joys of her youth when her twelve-year-old daughter started playing volleyball.

However, after a few attempts at helping her daughter practice in the backyard, "Sorry, honey, I can't," became a common, frustrating refrain, not just for her physical discomfort but for the moments lost with her daughter.

"Why won't this pain go away?" was a common question repeating in her mind as she stared at the ceiling while trying to drift off to sleep as the aching in her knee continued relentlessly, like the ticking of a clock echoing in the silence. No number of TikTok videos or Instagram reels, listening to meditation music, or counting sheep was able to distract her from the persistent ache that pulsed inside her knee, night after night.

Jean's journey through the maze of treatments—expensive programs that ended up being empty promises, cortisone injections offering fleeting solace, and medications that clouded more than just pain—had led her to my doorstep. Rather than a step toward healing, each intervention felt like a deeper entrenchment into despair. Her knee, once a source of strength, had become a constant reminder of her limitations, described by her doctor as "bone on bone," with surgery looming large as the only visible escape.

> **"Bone on bone" refers to the spaces within the joint narrowing to the point that they are almost rubbing on each other.**

Yet, Jean's resilience shone through. Her refusal to accept surgery as the sole solution was not born of denial, but of a deep belief that there had to be another way. A way that did not just silence the pain temporarily but addressed its roots, allowing her not just to dream of playing volleyball with her daughter or pickleball with her friends, but to make it a reality.

If you find yourself resonating with Jean's journey, feeling overwhelmed and lost in the endless sea of internet searches for the best braces, procedures, supplements, or remedies for relief, know that your struggle is shared by countless others. Consider the vast industry solely dedicated to supports and braces for pain; it soared to a $4 billion market in 2023. And when we factor in the market for pain-relieving medications, this number is anticipated to burgeon to nearly $116 billion by 2032, it's evident that the quest for alleviating pain is a widespread concern reaching epidemic proportions.

In the pages that follow, we embark on a journey to unravel the mysteries of the pain you are experiencing. We provide the foundation for insights that empower you to navigate a disheartening journey you did not sign up for and find the shift you need to finally get rid of your pain, or at the very least minimize it so it doesn't interfere with your daily life.

The Purpose of Pain

Understanding the true purpose of pain is pivotal as we embark on this journey to alleviate it.

Pain, at its core, is your body's ally, not its enemy.

I know how counterintuitive that might sound, especially when you're in the throes of discomfort that seems anything but protective. The sentiment, "I just can't live like this anymore!" or the desperate plea, "I just want it to stop so I can exercise, lose weight, and feel healthy" are complaints I hear often. Yet, if we pause for a moment to decode the message pain is sending us, we unlock the first clue in a mystery that many, like you, have been trying to solve through a myriad of remedies—each promising relief, yet often leading to a cabinet full of half-used supplements, a history of fleeting treatments, and a laundry list of medications that carry their own set of drawbacks. This conventional cycle, as you have probably found out, is focused solely on silencing symptoms and rarely leads to liberation.

Pain Is Your Protector, Not Your Adversary

Let's break it down:

Picture a typical Saturday morning. If you have had kids or have taken care of other kids, you might remember that it's likely earlier than you'd prefer to be awake, yet there you are in the kitchen with a curious toddler who has way too much energy for this time of day. While you prepare your hot coffee or tea, driven by curiosity, that miniature human reaches for something on a hot stove. The instant scream that follows captures your full attention, propelling you into action. Thankfully, the little red-eyed darling pulled her finger away before the skin was charred.

This scenario, fraught with fear and quick responses, illustrates pain's primal role: to signal danger and protect us from harm.

As you pull that little innocent darling away from the stove and give her a stern look, you might say, "No honey, that's hot!"

Then tears start to stream down her rosy cheeks, and you pull her in close, feeling your rapid heart rates reverberating together. In the heat of the moment, it's unlikely you're reflecting on the silver lining. Yet, there's an undeniable lesson. Her ability to feel pain, a natural guardian, spared her from a potentially severe burn. This moment, steeped in fear and quick action, underscores the invaluable lesson our body's pain response teaches us—it can keep us away from further harm.

Pain's messages, although sometimes harsh and unwelcome, are rooted in preservation. It's a system honed over millennia, designed to alert us to harm and urge us to take corrective action. It's why a sudden sharp pain in your back when bending over can immobilize you, as it did with a patient of mine named Steve.

Steve's Early Morning Wake-Up Call

The first hint of dawn was just peeking through the curtains when the piercing sound of the alarm jolted Steve awake. He lay there for a moment, gathering his thoughts and bracing himself for the day. As he swung his legs over the side of the bed, a gentle stiffness whispered through his lower back—a sign of yesterday's long hours at his desk. It was nothing out of the ordinary, just the usual reminder that he wasn't as young as he used to be.

With a quiet sigh, Steve stretched his arms over his head, feeling the familiar slight cramp between his shoulder blades. The room was still in the soft grip of morning, his slippers waiting patiently by the bed but just out of reach of his extended leg. So, he bent forward to grab them, a routine movement. In an instant, a sharp, stabbing pain exploded in his lower back, fierce and unforgiving. It seized his back and midsection like a vise grip. His hand slammed onto his wooden bedside table to give him some stability to ease the pain and keep him from sliding off the bed and falling to his knees.

Frozen, Steve inched his hand along the table that bore his full weight, his other hand pressing hard against his lower back. The pain radiated like wildfire, flaring out to his hip and down his leg, anchoring him in place with its fierce intensity. The room, so familiar and safe, spun slightly as he tried to straighten up, each movement igniting fresh sparks of agony.

Minutes passed like hours as Steve cautiously tested his body's limits, trying to find a way to stand up fully or lie down without excruciating pain. But every attempt was met with a harsh rebuke from his back. The searing pain was his beacon in the early morning, warning him to stop moving or further damage would result.

Defeated, he groaned and fell onto his elbow and then his side, picking up one leg, then the other, carefully positioning himself to minimize the pain.

As the initial wave of pain settled into a dull roar, Steve's thoughts turned grim. What if this wasn't just a simple strain like in the past? What if he couldn't get up to shower, go to work, or couldn't drive?

After ten to twenty minutes on his side, the pain subsided to a dull ache in his hip and top half of his buttock. After looking at his phone, he knew he would have to forgo his shower if he was going to make it to work on time. After gingerly putting on his clothes and grabbing his morning coffee, his small steps took him to his car. He slowly turned to his side and tried to pick up his leg to no avail. He had to back in, and as he settled behind the steering wheel to drive to work, the pain traveled down from his hip once again into his calf and foot. As the realization came to him that he would never be able to sit through eight hours of work, Steve found himself driving straight to the nearest urgent care.

A two-hour wait ensued. Steve underwent x-rays that turned up negative for any type of fracture, and was given temporary pain management—muscle relaxants and a strong anti-inflammatory—as well as his marching orders to fill his prescriptions at the local pharmacy. The medications promised relief, and at first, they seemed to deliver. He slept for what seemed like hours, and when he awakened, he could move again. The drugs masked the pain enough to function. But as the days and weeks went by, the relief came at a price. The drugs blurred the edges of his days, leaving him foggy and disconnected. The pain, dulled by chemicals, lingered as a constant undercurrent; a reminder that it was still there, waiting.

As weeks turned into months, Steve found himself wrestling with a tough decision. The medications made life bearable, but at what cost? His thoughts were no longer sharp and his mood was often as grey as the overcast skies of his Midwest morning commute.

One sleepless night, after months of taking the medications, while he lay awake listening to the rhythm of his labored breathing, Steve realized something had to change. He needed more than pills; he needed a new way forward.

This realization marked the beginning of Steve's true journey—a journey not just to treat pain, but to understand its messages and reclaim his life from its grasp. It was a path that would lead him through uncertainty and discovery, but one that held the promise of real, lasting change.

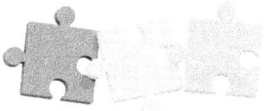

Key Pieces

Pain as a Protector: Pain is not your enemy; it's your body's way of signaling danger and preventing further harm. Understanding this is the first step toward managing and alleviating pain.

The Purpose of Pain: Pain serves as an essential warning system. It's a protective mechanism designed to prompt corrective action and prevent further injury.

The Conventional Approach Falls Short: Traditional treatments, like medication and injections, often focus on masking pain rather than addressing its root cause. These interventions can lead to temporary relief at times, but don't provide a long-term solution.

A New Path Forward: The journey to overcoming pain involves not just treating symptoms but understanding and addressing the underlying causes. This approach promises more than just temporary relief—it offers a chance to reclaim your life.

Pain, though unwelcome and, well ... painful, is a warning. It's a message from your body that sometimes speaks to you in whispers, but when ignored enough times, it will end up feeling like a brick to your forehead, stopping you in your tracks if that's what it takes to get your attention.

CHAPTER 2

Wired For Warning: How Pain Works

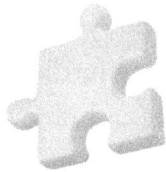

"Pain changes your life forever. But so does healing from it."

–Author unknown

Chuck sat in my office, his face etched with agony. He had recently twisted his ankle while playing soccer with his son, and the sharp pain had been immediate and intense. After he took his shoe off, he reported that "it swelled up like a balloon."

Chuck's experience was a classic case of acute pain—sudden, sharp, and ultimately, after our treatment that day, short-lived. As we discussed in Chapter 1, this pain was the body's way of signaling an injury and prompting immediate immobilization to prevent further damage. With time and proper treatment, his ankle would heal in a few short weeks and the pain would likely disappear.

Over the course of three treatments that he needed on his ankle, we continued our conversation, and Chuck, like many of the forty-plus-year-olds that I see in my clinic, spoke of another area of pain that had plagued him for many years. This one had become a constant presence in his life. "I've had this lower back pain for years," he admitted. "Some days it's a dull ache, other days it's a sharp, shooting pain. It never really goes away."

The Tale of Two Pain Types

No matter who you are, your body functions very similarly to every other human. The body is an intricate symphony of cells, nerves, organs, and tissues, all interconnected by a vast network of communication channels. Your kidneys are a filtering machine. Your liver helps you with digestion and getting rid of toxins, and your heart pumps blood through your body sixty to one hundred times a minute. I could go on and on with each body part and what it does, but I think you get the point. Therefore, at the very basic level of understanding, as discussed in the last chapter, pain is part of the body's grand plan. It's the most annoying note in the body's symphony.

We tend to want to cover it up so we can ignore it and continue on with our day. But in truth, it should not be shrouded or neglected, as it is the crucial response designed to protect you from potential danger or further injury.

1.   Acute Pain: The Body's Immediate Response

In the case of Chuck's sprained ankle, this was an example of acute pain. Though there's definitely nothing 'cute' about it in any way, shape, or form, it is usually resolved rather quickly. The pain experienced, however, is valuable as the body's rapid response system to detect and avoid danger.

This response can certainly come in handy throughout our lives. Take, for example, people in the world born with rare genetic diseases that result in not feeling pain, which at first glance probably sounds like heaven. But those who have these types of disorders, such as Congenital Insensitivity to Pain with Anhidrosis (CIPA), who don't have a protective pain response because they were born without the much-needed connection between pain-sensing nerves and the brain, don't typically live past twenty-five years old.

For the vast majority of people who can feel pain, this "gift" has allowed us to survive throughout the years. Here's how it works.

PAIN 101

The body employs specialized sensors at the end of nerves to detect various types of signals transmitted by chemicals crossing the space between the nerves. These spaces are called synapses.

Think of nerves as long cables that act like extension cords coming from the brain. They connect almost at their ends but not quite. Instead, a synapse or space exists between them. Chemicals travel across the synapses from one nerve ending to another, and this initiates another signal being sent down the next cord (nerve). But instead of sending signals only one way, there's a two-way track in these nerves that go to and from the brain via the spinal cord.

At the end of the nerves, within the synapses where the chemicals are released, are sensors called receptors.

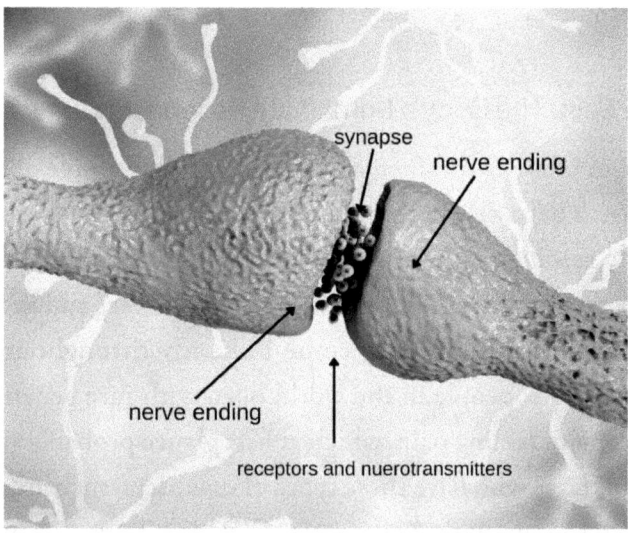

Figure 2.1 Two nerve endings connecting, and neurotransmitters being released into the synapse. This release and stimulation of the receptors results in communication that creates the next action potential/nerve impulse to travel down or up the nerve on the right and deliver its message.

Types of Receptors

- Pain receptors (nociceptors) are akin to an alarm system warning you of danger.
- Thermoreceptors (detecting temperature) can be compared to a temperature sensor in a computer, monitoring the device's heat level. Remember our toddler in the kitchen? Pain appears when the temperature sensors get too hot.
- Mechanoreceptors (detecting pressure and vibration) are like keyboard keys that respond to touch. They lie within the skin and help us detect pressure and vibration and help us differentiate between what is harmful or benign.

These sensors/receptors between nerves can identify whether you are experiencing mechanical forces like pressure, temperature changes, and even changes inside the body resulting from inflammation, or outside the body from external irritants like chemicals or heat.

Imagine the pain associated with dropping a weight on your foot during a workout or while cleaning out your garage. The result? You end up hopping around on one foot like someone gone rogue in a hopscotch competition. This is an example of the mechanical pain receptors in your foot instantly springing into action.

They generate electrical signals that travel along your nerves, reaching your spinal cord. At the spinal cord and between nerves, these signals trigger the release of neurotransmitters (chemicals) that cross the connection between nerves to create yet another electrical impulse. This electrical impulse continues to travel up the spine and along other nerves toward the brain. See Figure 2.2

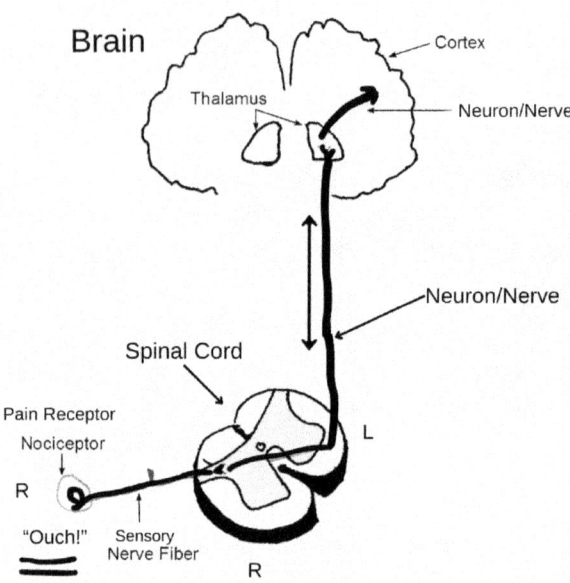

Figure 2.2 Nerve transmission from nociceptor (pain receptor) to spinal cord to brain

Faster than we can blink an eye, the impulse will ping nerve receptors in the brain, resulting in not only telling us that we have pain, but also sending signals to the muscles in our legs to keep the weight off that injured foot to prevent further injury. At times, the signal can just ping off the spinal cord and avoid traveling all the way to the brain. This is sometimes referred to as a 'no brainer,' and we react with a reflex resulting in avoidance of the pain.

This immediate reaction, without conscious thought, is an excellent example of the body's protective mechanism. This is acute pain. This type of pain represents damage to the tissues and recruits the body's own healing mechanisms to take care of it, eventually returning our tissue to its normal state within a few days or weeks. Hopefully, this results in us being a bit more careful with a dumbbell the next time.

Acute Pain:

- Happens suddenly
- Starts out sharp or intense
- Initiates inflammation
- Healing process begins
- Tissue is healed and pain goes away in a few days to a few weeks

2. Chronic Pain: When the Alarm Bells Keep Ringing

Chronic pain, on the other hand, is a different story.

Joy lay in bed staring at her phone, scrolling through endless images consisting not only of the best meal her friends just ate, but of them having fun and smiling at their different family events or playing with their kids or grandkids. Her eyes welled up and her chest tightened a bit. It had been almost a year since Joy had been able to experience anything she would describe as "fun."

Her eyes traveled to the clock on her phone. It read 2:54 a.m. She had been awakened yet again by the constant aching in her shoulder. The pain had resulted in her not being able to go to her friend's son's wedding. She wanted to avoid all the questions about where she had been and the unsolicited advice about what she should do about her neck and shoulder.

Joy had declined the offer to join her friends on a walk so many times in the previous six months that they stopped asking her to come along. It was a good hour of her being awake before she started to feel sleepy again. She thought the medications, which she knew weren't great for her stomach, had finally started to kick in.

Joy knew her options, according to her doctor: surgery or more injections, and she just wasn't ready to do either.

Chronic Pain

- Continues for more than three months
- Can be sharp, dull, aching, burning, etc.
- May involve inflammation, or the tissue can look perfectly normal
- Healing process is stuck
- Pain continues to be triggered

Why Can't I Turn Off the Alarm?

Chronic pain, pain that lasts for more than three months, resulted in Joy's decreased activity and the beginning of her social isolation. Steve, whose back injury was described in Chapter One, decided to finally do something different after yet another sleepless night. Due to the chronic back pain, he had been using his vacation days because he just couldn't sit at his desk for eight hours a day. His duties at work were limited, and his employers were getting more and more frustrated with him.

At our appointment, Steve told me his doctor went over his MRI results and told him it showed some degeneration in his spine that could be part of the issue. But he was told by his first orthopedic doctor that he wasn't a candidate for surgery. He was partly relieved not to have surgery, but another part of him was disappointed, as he was hoping for a solution to the ongoing pain.

Twelve months after the initial injury, he continued to feel pain despite the muscle relaxants, steroids, anti-inflammatories, and the nerve and pain medications. Because the pain did not resolve, he told the third orthopedic doctor he couldn't live with the pain the way it was. Steve put on thirty pounds, drank too much alcohol, and stopped going out with friends. Despite only mild disc bulging noted on the MRI, Steve ended up going to another doctor and having a laminectomy, a surgical procedure where surgeons remove a part of the vertebrae (the bones stacked on one another in the spine) to make more room for the nerves that come off the spinal cord. If the bulging discs were putting pressure on the nerve, the goal was to eliminate the pressure and, hopefully, the accompanying symptoms. But unfortunately for Steve, the surgery resulted in more time off but no significant relief months after surgery.

Jean, who you met at the beginning of the book, with a 'bone on bone' description of her knee from her doctor, was experiencing chronic pain, as well. Her pain was impacting her work and quality time with her daughter, as well as social activities, but she wanted to avoid surgery because her mom had a knee replacement that did not provide the relief it had promised, and she did not want to go through the same thing. She dreaded every step up or down stairs that she had to take because pain would shoot down from the inside of her knee to the inside of her leg. Other times, the knee just burned, even when she was sitting or had the leg elevated in her recliner at home.

Joy, Steve, and Jean were continually prescribed pain meds and anti-inflammatories starting when they had mild pain, all the way through and beyond when their pain became chronic. Sometimes, but not always, prescriptions are combined with physical or occupational therapy, and while some people achieve relief, many are still stuck months and years later on a life-altering journey where there is no end in sight.

Does Chronic Pain Have a Purpose?

Remember how we discussed that acute pain has a purpose to protect us? We tend to forget or don't even consider that the same is true for chronic pain.

How in the world does chronic pain protect you? To those who suffer from it, they would gladly go without such protection if that meant relief, and that is why medication after medication are utilized to cover up the pain.

But consider this: instead of covering up the pain from the beginning like an overprotective parent who wants their child to avoid any suffering at all costs and typically winds up being detrimental to the child in the long run, what can happen when we see pain for what it really is: our protector? It's the body's constant effort to help us keep from hurting ourselves further.

Unfortunately, we have been conditioned to think of chronic pain, or any pain for that matter, as something to cover up instead of listening to whatever it is trying to tell us. Chronic pain often results from attempts to place a gag order over the pain that we have experienced in the past.

We think of pain as nature's cruel joke that we want to get rid of as soon as possible instead of what it actually is: a phenomenal mechanism our body uses to get our attention and keep us safe from harm now or in the future. It's a signal to be listened to and learned from, but even intelligent and extremely knowledgeable experts think of some mechanisms of pain as malicious pranks our body is playing on us.

Dr. Peter Attia, author of the book *Outlive*, had guest Dr. Stuart McGill on his podcast, where they had an in-depth discussion about back pain. Dr. McGill is an esteemed professor emeritus from the University of Waterloo and holds the position of chief scientific officer at Backfitpro.com. His expertise centers on analyzing intricate lower back pain cases from around the world. Dr. McGill's work is groundbreaking and should be mainstream. I loved all the detail he went into during Dr. Attia's nearly three-hour podcast.

When repetitive trauma or shearing forces occur from incorrect movement patterns, or not enough stability or flexibility, an intervertebral disc (the structural shock absorbers between each vertebra in the spine) can become injured. Dr. McGill explained that when an injured disc can't maintain the shock absorption like it used to, the gel-like material protrudes from the middle of the disc (see Figure 2.3). It pushes through different layers of tissue or structures called annular rings (similar to the circles you would see on a tree stump after the tree has been cut down) meant to protect and conserve its shock absorbing ability. This can result in what doctors call a bulging, or eventually, a herniated disc. Interestingly enough, in a true herniation, this protrusion will be the first time this gel-like substance comes in direct contact with the body's immune system.

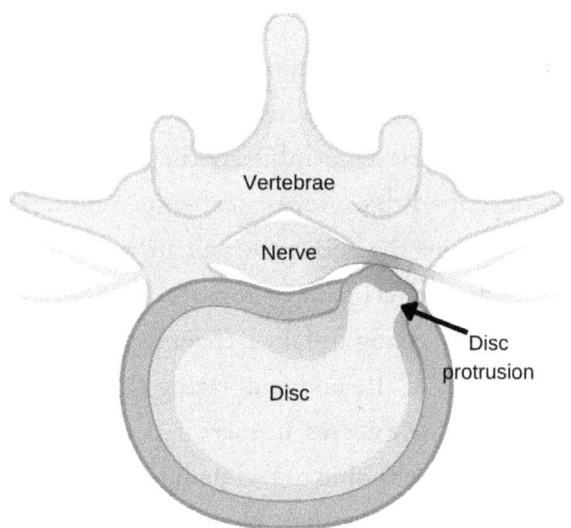

Figure 2.3 A gel-like inner part of a disc protruding and putting pressure on a nerve.

This new exposure to the immune system creates a reaction that causes significant inflammation in the area. The resulting pain can be in one spot or shoot down the extremity, or possibly skip the arm or leg and be felt far away from the infraction, i.e., in the hands or feet. It can be debilitating. Steve, our example earlier in the chapter, knows this feeling all too well.

At the time of this infarction, the disc is not able to maintain the high pressure of the once-effective shock absorption system. Now, like a small pinhole puncture in a balloon, that balloon (or in this case, the disc) loses some or all of its pressure or ability to absorb shock, according to Dr. McGill. And due to this injury, nerves and blood vessels start to grow within the disc for the very first time. These nerves, specifically, now allow you to feel pain near (or far from) the area of injury. This is why, as the disc breaks through or stretches the aforementioned annular rings (which can take months or even years), you do not feel pain. It was because there were no nerves present in those tissues until, of course, you experienced the straw that broke the camel's back. In Steve's case, that was when he bent over to pick up his slippers. This movement either pushed the gel out past its last ring or stretched the last ring far enough outside its original position to irritate or infiltrate the area around the nerve.

Dr. McGill described this process as being "unfair." He said, "You damage the disc and now the body grows a hardware (nerves and blood vessels) inside the disc to feel pain even more." Attia agreed.

However, instead of being unfair, I encourage you to think of this process as another one of the body's amazing capabilities. It truly is a brilliant mechanism. Those nerves, now created as a result of injury, will cause pain where we weren't able to feel pain before. Had we been able to feel pain months or years earlier when the annular rings were first breached, we may have done something sooner to prevent the progressive damage. But the body, by design, bought us time before we experienced pain's debilitating outcome.

When we finally feel pain, our body sends us a signal to say, "There's something wrong here, don't move further." It is our alarm system signaling caution ahead. If we continue to ignore that alarm system by covering it up with medications, or we keep moving, lifting, and twisting improperly without creating stability to protect this now-vulnerable area, we blow through our warning system like a car running a red light, and sooner or later, if that continues, a much more serious injury occurs.

Don't get me wrong, I LOVE Peter Attia's podcast, and I hope you listen to this informative talk with Dr. McGill. I am in awe of the information that both Dr. McGill and Dr. Attia put out into the world, but their conversation and take on pain as being "unfair" is a perfect example of how even highly-intelligent, open-minded, evidence-based scholars have been conditioned to automatically describe the body's natural protective process as something negative, i.e., something to be frustrated by and cause us to think our body has failed us when in fact it's simply protecting us.

Now let's see how we can leverage the body's innate intelligence behind pain to resolve it.

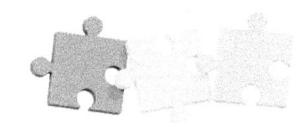

Key Pieces

Acute Pain vs. Chronic Pain: Acute pain is the body's immediate response to injury, serving as a protective mechanism to prevent further damage. Chronic pain, lasting more than three months, is more complex and often indicates underlying issues that need to be addressed.

The Body's Pain Mechanism: Pain signals are transmitted through specialized sensors (receptors) in the body, which detect mechanical forces, temperature changes, and inflammation. These signals travel to the brain, triggering responses to protect the body from harm.

Pain as a Warning: Acute and chronic pain is the body's way of signaling that something is wrong. It's not just an inconvenience, but instead serves as a vital message that should not be continually ignored or simply masked with medications.

Understanding Pain's Purpose: Pain, whether acute or chronic, is a protective mechanism designed by the body to alert us to danger and guide us toward healing. Misinterpreting or ignoring these signals can lead to more significant issues down the road.

Common Misconceptions About Pain: Even experts sometimes view pain as an unfortunate consequence rather than recognizing its role as a crucial protective mechanism. Embracing pain as a guide rather than an adversary is essential for long-term healing.

CHAPTER 3

What Your Doctor May Not Have Told You About the Conventional Treatment of Your Pain

"Conformity means following the crowd down conventional paths and maintaining the status quo. Originality is taking the road less traveled, championing a set of novel ideas that go against the grain but ultimately make things better."

–*Author Adam Grant*

While I was on the dance floor enjoying the parental responsibility of teaching my then-twenty-two-year-old son how to properly polka, the sudden 'pop' in my knee was followed by what I could only describe as a hot poker being shoved between my femur and tibia. This resulted in massive swelling and pain so severe, as you read in the introduction, I couldn't bear weight without feeling as though glass shards were penetrating my knee joint.

You have probably had a similar feeling of intense pain at some point in your life, whether it was a back that seized up or a joint that experienced a sharp jolt with a quick twist, or a cramp while you were trying to reach or pick up something.

Whatever the event, if you are reading this book, you have likely been stopped in your tracks or sidelined due to a sudden injury that came out of nowhere. What followed was an intricate process that your body performs every millisecond of every day, one of which you are mostly unaware of until something sudden and painful happens.

This experience results in inflammation.

Inflammation: Friend or Foe?

With the experience of acute pain, inflammation is always the culprit. And in many cases, inflammation plays a significant role in the chronic joint or muscle pain you may be experiencing now.

But what is inflammation exactly? Is it truly all bad?

Why is it important that our medical system acknowledges it? And why is it that the quick fixes usually prescribed by those solely sticking to the conventional medicine approach or available over the counter may not be the best option for pain in the short or long run?

Anti-Inflammatories in the Good Ol' Days

When I earned my first college degree, which my son thinks was back in the horse-drawn carriage era, we learned about inflammation. Most of what we learned about in the nineties could be summed up in one thought: inflammation was bad. Or at least that is how I remembered it. It was something we wanted to get rid of quickly.

RICE was and still is a popular acronym for what you should do to get rid of inflammation after an injury.

Rest
Ice
Compression
Elevation

This advice still has its merits, especially in the acute phase of injuries, when swelling and pain are still present. What is not present in that acronym, however, is today's typical response to pain: medication.

The Rise of Anti-Inflammatory Medications

As more drugs called nonsteroidal anti-inflammatories (NSAIDs) became available, both by prescription and over the counter, physicians began recommending them more frequently, and pharmaceutical companies increased direct-to-consumer advertising more significantly. Patients, in turn, started buying and using them more for themselves and their families.

Direct To Consumer Advertising Spend By Pharmaceutical Companies

Advertising from pharmaceutical companies direct to consumer (DTCA) became extremely popular in the early 90s. Pharmaceutical industry spending on this type of advertising rose from $55 million in 1991 to $363 million in 1995. In 1997, the FDA relaxed the requirements for the pharmaceutical industry's television broadcast advertising, and between 1997 and 1998, spending from drug companies on DTCA on television doubled to $664 million, and this amount skyrocketed to $3.3 billion by 2005, and $6 billion by 2016. And though in 2023, television broadcasting commercials from the pharmaceutical industry stayed steady at approximately $6 billion dollars, the amount spent by pharma on digital advertising has soared to $14 billion. This is expected to reach $19 billion in 2024.

This trend became clear to me in the early 2000s during a trip back home from Australia. After deplaning in Los Angeles, I found myself on a crowded shuttle bus heading to the domestic terminal. The passengers, tired from a long thirteen-hour flight, were packed in, standing and sitting shoulder to shoulder.

Across from me, I noticed a young boy, his head buried in his hands. "It hurts," I heard him murmur to the woman beside him. "My head hurts."

The woman, who I assumed was his mother given their similar features, began rummaging through her purse. I heard the rattle of a bottle as she pulled it out, unscrewed the cap, and tapped out a tablet into her palm.

"Here, take this," she said, maneuvering her hand toward the boy.

"No, I don't want it," he replied, head resting in his hands.

"I said take it!" she insisted, her voice rising with frustration.

"No," he repeated, defiant.

The mother's patience waned. She pinched the boy's jacket sleeve with her other hand and nudged him toward her. Their eyes met, hers wide and intense. "Take it," she said, her voice low but deliberate.

The boy hesitated, then reluctantly took the pill from her hand and popped it in his mouth. She pulled a bottle of water from the backpack wedged between them and handed it to him as they both sat in silence.

As I watched this exchange, I couldn't help but think back to my own childhood decades before. If I had complained of a headache, my parents would have told me, "it will go away eventually," or simply told me to drink some water. Now, the quick fix—a pill to relieve both the boy's pain and his mother's worry—seemed to have become an everyday expectation. The contrast was stark, and the realization that this was our new normal settled heavily on me.

Numbers Don't Lie: Inflammation Is a Big Business

The numbers are clear. Along with the entire pharmaceutical industry advertising directly to consumers, the use of NSAIDs and opioids increased four-fold from 1996 to 2018. The market for these types of drugs is large and only expected to grow. Research in 2020 showed that the money made from nonsteroidal anti-inflammatories (NSAIDs) was $16.4 billion overall in the United States. That market is projected to boom to $28.6 billion by 2030.

Decreasing inflammation and pain with drugs has become commonplace, as well as a part of big business. But is it always the healthiest and best choice in the short and long term?

Short- and Long-Term Consequences of Taking NSAIDs

What are the consequences of using these anti-inflammatories, and what about the body's ability to decrease inflammation without outside assistance from a pill?

Granted, these medications seem to be beneficial at times. They appear to help us get rid of inflammation and pain quickly after an injury so we can be functional more quickly. But because of the prevalence of prescription writing for NSAIDs and the ease of grabbing anti-inflammatory medications off the shelf, we often forget or haven't been told how these drugs can impact what our body naturally can do. It is not often if ever discussed, except now in this book, that there is an increased risk of developing chronic pain for those taking NSAIDs in the acute phase of an injury.

Research shows that when the body's immune system and healing response is suppressed after the onset of acute pain, the person who takes anti-inflammatory drugs is more likely to develop chronic pain. The marketing of these drugs literally banks on this lack of knowledge and preference for convenience in the short term, instead of making customers aware of potential long-term consequences.

But what can consumers do? Some of my patients can't make it through the day or sleep at night if they don't take their medications. And most patients, when asked, would prefer to *not* have to continue taking the medications, and want information about alternatives to help them decrease or eliminate their reliance on them.

Therefore, to accomplish this, it's essential to learn about what inflammation is, if it's all bad, and how to address it to relieve the joint and muscle pain you are experiencing.

Inflammation: Is it All Bad?

When most people hear about inflammation these days, they assume it is all bad. Too much inflammation and chronic inflammation are not good things by any means, but inflammation is truly a process we literally can't live without. So, as much as the advertisers would like you to believe it's all bad, that is just not the truth.

Like pain, what if we started to think of some inflammation as a natural part of our healing process, to be paid attention to at times when we experience injury or pain, but not a terrible thing that needs to be snuffed out completely?

The fact is that we can't get rid of all inflammation, and honestly, we don't want to.

If we did not have inflammation, we would cease to exist very quickly. Inflammation is the body's best defense against illness, injuries, and infections (viral or bacterial). If we did not have inflammation as a defense against these events, we wouldn't be able to survive. Chronic inflammation, however, is another story, and thankfully, this can be avoided or addressed, but we will get to that later.

For now, understanding inflammation is essential to eventually getting rid of joint and muscle pain.

Inflammation 101

Several times a day, I have the following conversation in my office.

Me: With the treatment you are trialing today, our goal is to help your body increase its innate natural anti-inflammatory capabilities, and to help decrease or eliminate the pain you are experiencing.

Patient: Sounds good.

Me: Okay, inflammation is essential to our survival. It has three phases: the pro-inflammatory phase, the anti-inflammatory phase, and the healing or resolution phase.

Patient: Oh, so what phase am I in?

Me: Potentially, you are stuck in the pro-inflammatory phase.

Patient: Okay.

Me: Let's talk about how your body in general can move through that phase to get to healing.

When you scratch your hand, for example, it immediately gets red, warm, and puffy. That is the pro-inflammatory phase. This phase is chaotic with many substances heading toward the injured area to address the damage. This is much like the time right after a crash on the highway where people are gathering to see what happened, and first responders are heading to the scene. This pro-inflammatory phase develops quickly after an injury. It's why sometimes you feel that the area feels warm to the touch. When there is an injury, your body's white blood cells, or its first responders (think fire fighters and paramedics going to the accident), head over to the injury to start the repair process and attempt to minimize the damage.

Patient: Got it.

Me: When you leave that scratch alone for a few days (i.e., take the trigger of the inflammation away), you notice that the redness has gone down or disappeared; it's not as puffy anymore, but you can still see that it isn't fully healed yet. That's the anti-inflammatory phase.

In our car accident analogy, the cleanup crew (anti-inflammatory molecules) arrived after the emergency services (pro-inflammatory molecules) had dealt with the immediate threat. If you have ever seen pictures of what a car on fire on the highway looks like after the first responders have put out the blaze and tended to any injured party, you can visualize what a mess the injury and the first responders had to make. If that mess isn't cleaned up, if the debris isn't taken away, the traffic can't go back to normal, right?

Patient: That's right.

Me: Let's go back to that scratch on your hand. After a week or two, you can look at your hand, and there is no sign of that scratch. That shows that the tissue has healed at the surface, and if you touch it and it's sore, there might still be healing happening underneath the skin, but overall that injury is on its way to being entirely resolved. That is the resolution or healing phase.

It would be similar to restoring traffic to an orderly flow after the accident had been cleaned up and restored.

Patient: So, you are saying that my joint is stuck in the pro-inflammatory phase, but I have been taking anti-inflammatories. Shouldn't that have helped the process along?

Me: If you have been using anti-inflammatories after the initial injury or symptom, and when they wear off, the symptoms come back, it's not likely that the anti-inflammatories are helping you completely resolve the issue, and they may be causing more issues for you in the long run. Here is how they work.

How Nonsteroidal Anti-Inflammatories (NSAIDs) Work

Think of a bustling, busy metropolitan area like New York City. To keep people moving to their jobs and the other places they travel each day, there's a complex traffic signal system that controls the flow of transportation. Our complex system in the body is akin to that traffic system. Like the multiple pathways in the city, i.e., streets, alleys, and buildings in New York, we have pathways in our bodies that are made up of blood vessels, nerves, the lymph system, organs, and more.

Specifically, in the body, there is a pathway on which NSAIDs have their effect. It's called the arachidonic acid pathway. That's a mouthful, I agree. The arachidonic acid pathway, when functioning well, is like a complex system of highways and streets with the appropriate signals to slow, stop, or speed up the body's inflammatory cycle. Just like the traffic system in a big city, in the body, this pathway helps to ensure that when inflammation is created, it is eventually resolved, and the body continues to thrive.

But what happens when something breaks down and the system experiences some sort of alarming event?

The Incident:

One day, an accident (injury or infection) occurs on a main street or busy highway (a part of your body). The traffic signals (the arachidonic pathway) change color to adjust traffic and relay appropriate help (molecules related to inflammation) to the accident site. This can result in a traffic jam (pro-inflammatory stage) and detours—it's messy, but it's also necessary to address the incident and keep the rest of the system working.

Pro-inflammatory and Anti-inflammatory Signals:

The red and yellow signals and flashing lights on emergency vehicles ensure that first responders (immune cells and pro-inflammatory mediators) reach the site quickly to manage the crisis. Other police officers and city workers (anti-inflammatory mediators) are being summoned to go help with the eventual cleanup during and after everything has been stabilized.

Anti-inflammatory Drugs:

Imagine anti-inflammatory drugs (e.g., NSAIDs) as FBI agents descending on the scene from out of town to assist traffic cops, city workers, or engineers whom the body naturally has sent to the scene to stabilize it and then clean it up. We've all seen that movie. These FBI agents manually override the signals as well as the local police officers, and they take control of the scene. They force the reduction of first responders and red and yellow signals (pro-inflammatory molecules) faster than normal, allowing traffic to flow more freely and faster, thereby reducing the bottleneck (inflammation). Suppose the accident is small enough and there aren't too many other accidents in the city. In that case, this extra help from the FBI (NSAIDs) for a short period can get everything running and back to normal faster (tissue heals, pain is gone).

However, if after the FBI agents leave, or in other words, your anti-inflammatory medications wear off before healing can occur or overstay their welcome, stay too long, i.e., there aren't enough first responders or any local police around anymore, another bottleneck of traffic or another accident occurs (inflammation and its symptoms return).

If you repeat the cycle with more and more anti-inflammatory medications and then continue to irritate the tissue with movement because you don't feel pain anymore, the body's natural inflammatory cycle can't run its course, and may start over again and again, or never get resolved. This is one way that chronic pain can result.

The FBI agents (NSAIDs) may sound like a good idea because they helped the symptoms resolve quickly. But when used frequently, they may be creating more harm than good, interfering with the body's natural protective mechanism and, subsequently, its ability to heal.

Pills: Quick Fixes with Long-Term Consequences

Oftentimes, patients ask my opinion of whether they should keep taking NSAIDs, get a cortisone injection, or take a stronger oral anti-inflammatory like meloxicam or prednisone. My answer is always, "That's up to you and your prescribing doctor," since every person should make the choice that is best for them. But a typical conversation may go like this:

Patient: Okay, now I understand that the medications (nonsteroidal anti-inflammatories) may not be the best thing to stop the inflammation fully right after I am injured because they interfere with the body's natural healing process, but someone told me to keep taking them to stay ahead of the pain and inflammation. So, if I keep taking them (NSAIDs), won't they just knock the inflammation out once and for all?

Me: That would seem like a great idea. If, in some circumstances, NSAIDs can help at the beginning, why shouldn't you just keep taking them, because it would make sense that you want to limit or stop inflammation to take away the pain?

In the example I gave above, we talked about the FBI agents (NSAIDs) taking over for the local authorities and city workers (natural anti-inflammatories). Based on research about these medications, it seems that this isn't such a good idea in the short or long term. Preventing or slowing our body's natural healing process by taking these pills right away could have consequences that can be detrimental not only to the area intended to be healed but also to other parts and processes of the body.

In a study of nearly one hundred patients with low back pain after an injury, researchers noticed that when the injured people took NSAIDs, there was a reduction of a type of white blood cell called neutrophils. They found that the human subjects who took NSAIDs early on for their pain tended to develop chronic back pain more often. Therefore, the pain-reducing effects of the medications in the short term may be setting people up for increased pain in the long term.

Another way of looking at this using our analogy of the traffic jam after an accident would be when the FBI agents (NSAIDs) came in to take over for the first responders and block out the city workers and police, this may have slowed or stopped the response of an important component of restoring order and function. Let's call the local law enforcement and city workers neutrophils. These cells come to clean up and help restore normal function in an area of the body that has been injured or irritated. Without these innate substances, it seems that what was once an organized flow with only occasional minor issues can become a chronic, persistent issue since the natural fixers (the neutrophils), part of the body's own healing process, were slowed down or stopped and debris and other irritants may still remain, causing the inflammatory reaction to come back and never resolve.

That is great news for the company selling the drugs. They have a long-term customer. But it's not great news for the people taking them.

Therefore, what you might think you are doing to help your pain in the short term is potentially setting you up for more pain in the long term.

> Let the body do its thing and seek help to assess the situation. When there is a non-life-threatening injury, let the natural healing process get started, and then you can control the swelling locally with RICE (i.e. rest, ice, compression, elevation), previously discussed. Yes, this process is longer and may seem inconvenient in the short term, but it's much more effective, efficient, and streamlined when the body has what it needs to complete the process on its own.
> Part 2 of this book is dedicated to helping you give your body what it needs to complete the process of healing.

As a result of the FBI agents or NSAIDs coming in and disrupting the normal flow of how things are handled, other issues start to pop up. These are side effects. When you stop a natural process of the body, another or several processes have to adjust, as well. This creates relatively common side effects of most medications (i.e., gastrointestinal irritation) resulting in:

- Indigestion
- Diarrhea
- Headaches

Or less common side effects from longer-term use:

- Kidney Dysfunction

- Heart Failure
- Heart Attacks
- Strokes

List of which anti-inflammatory drugs are commonly used for joint and muscle pain.
Common nonprescription-strength NSAIDs include:

- Aspirin (Bayer®, St. Joseph®)
- Ibuprofen (Motrin®, Advil®)
- Naproxen sodium (Aleve®)

Some of the most common prescription-strength NSAIDs include:

- Celecoxib (Celebrex®)
- Diclofenac (Voltaren®)
- Fenoprofen (Nalfon®)
- Indomethacin (Indocin®)
- Ketorolac (Toradol®)
- Meloxicam (Mobic)

Corticosteroid Injections: Is Cortisone Good or Bad?

Patient: What about cortisone injections? My doctor suggested I get a cortisone injection in my joint if the pain doesn't go away.

Me: Remember that pathway that we talked about previously, the arachidonic acid pathway? It's the pathway that acts like a traffic signaling system that controls traffic flow and responds to emergencies. When the body is disturbed due to an accident or injury, it sends the first responders (pro-inflammatory molecules) and then its local police and city workers (anti-inflammatory molecules like neutrophils) to get things cleaned up and resolved so traffic can flow normally again (tissue healing).

Cortisone and other drugs such as prednisone are classified as corticosteroids. Instead of being like FBI agents (NSAIDs) that take over and eliminate city workers and police officers. (first responders) They act more like a flame retardant that is dumped from a helicopter or plane over a fire that is burning out of control. These drugs douse the flame from above and stop all the (immune systems) first responders. In our accident analogy, the corticosteroids stops or significantly slows down the police, ambulances, city workers, onlookers (come on, you know you've slowed down to take a peek at an accident), and other supporting-cast members from getting to the area. Cortisone knocks out the pathway at a higher level and stops or slows down both the body's natural PRO-inflammatory molecules that cause the pain, redness, and swelling *and* the ANTI-inflammatory molecules that do the cleanup and allow tissue repair at a higher level than the NSAIDs. Therefore, the injection of cortisone can work like a charm to get rid of pain locally if they are injected into exactly the right place and systemically if prednisone is taken orally. But research shows that knocking out the body's natural inflammatory process with these corticosteroids (cortisone, prednisone, hydrocortisone), whether they are taken by mouth or injected locally has significant longer-term consequences.

More research is being done to assess the extent of this, but starting in 2017-2018, studies have confirmed the association of cortisone injections with negative side effects in joints. These include:

- Accelerated arthritis progression
- Stress fracture that occurs just beneath the cartilage in a joint
- Faster joint deterioration
- Bone death

In the shoulder, cortisone injections have been associated with a seven-times greater risk of rotator cuff tendon tears after the injection.

In addition, when over 10,000 individuals fifty years or older were assessed after a cortisone injection for a joint issue, a small but clinically significant result showed an increased risk of acute coronary syndrome (a sudden reduction of blood flow to the heart caused by a blockage) within a week of having the injection.

So, what was once considered a helpful, simple procedure for quick and potentially lasting pain relief should now be reconsidered due to its potential long-term and short-term side effects. Unfortunately, despite this evidence, cortisone injections are still given regularly, mainly because they are, as of this writing, still covered by insurance.

> **Another vote against cortisone injections:**
> In one study that looked at over 400 individuals who had cortisone injections, researchers found that a year later, the pain and stiffness in their joints had increased and their physical functioning was worse than those who had joint pain but did not get the injections.

Oral Corticosteroids

Oral corticosteroids, drugs such as Prednisone taken by mouth, inhibit the arachidonic acid pathway throughout the whole body. In other words, they address inflammation not simply in one spot, but around the entire body. Now that you know all inflammation isn't bad, and we need the inflammatory process for healing, you can understand why long-term use of these medications is less than ideal.

When these corticosteroids are taken by mouth, they pass through the stomach and intestine before entering the bloodstream, where they have systemic effects. But because they too are stopping many natural processes in the body, they also have multiple systemic side effects, especially when taken for extended periods. These can include:

- Weight gain and fluid retention
- Increased blood sugar (hyperglycemia)
- Osteoporosis
- Suppression of the immune system
- Insomnia, mood swings, or psychological effects
- Increased risk of infections
- Adrenal suppression (reduced production of natural cortisol by the adrenal glands)

Patient: Okay, I get it. Anti-inflammatories and cortisone injections can slow down the body's natural healing process, but what about Tylenol? Is it safe to take to decrease inflammation and reduce pain?

Pain and Fever Reliever

Me: Great question. But first, we have to clarify something. Tylenol (Acetaminophen) is not an anti-inflammatory medication. Instead, it's used as a pain reliever and an anti-pyretic, meaning besides relieving pain, it can help to reduce fever.

Both pain and fever are messages from the body. However, out of the scope of muscle and joint pain, keep in mind that having a fever is a sign that the body's natural healing process is working. The body is trying to fight the infection. And there are mixed opinions on whether fevers should be suppressed unless they are at dangerous levels. Relating this to our discussion on joint and muscle pain, however, acetaminophen does not reduce inflammation in joints, but it will in some cases decrease pain.

Patient: How does Tylenol work?
Me: Another great question! Even though it's been used since 1955, there is still some confusion as to how, exactly, Tylenol works to reduce pain.

The theories consist of the following:

1. Tylenol could have an impact on substances in the brain called COX 3 (part of that arachidonic pathway), which could reduce other substances called prostaglandins. Therefore, Tylenol may contribute to a numbing or analgesic effect.
2. Some research says that Tylenol may work on the endocannabinoid system, the same system that cannabinoids (i.e., THC/marijuana) influence. This system helps to reduce pain.
3. Other studies reveal a possible connection to serotonin, a chemical that influences mood, but also our perception of pain.

Basically, Tylenol may work on the brain's response to pain, potentially blocking signals that would tell us that we have pain. It doesn't impact what is causing the pain, i.e., the root cause of the pain, but it can help people avoid feeling it.

Patient: Is it safe to take for chronic pain?

Me: It really depends on the situation. A 2019 review of the existing literature revealed that although frequently prescribed for chronic pain from osteoarthritis, the evidence is scarce.

Tylenol (Acetaminophen) is often touted as one of the safest drugs on the market. However, if the powers that be aren't sure how it works, and they don't know exactly what it is doing in the body, then I am not sure they can definitively say it is safe. My guess is that *if* more research goes into trying to identify more side effects of Tylenol, since it's so widely used, they will see more side effects linked to it.

For example, in February 2022, the University of Edinburgh published a study. It found that a group of 110 patients with a history of high blood pressure saw an increase in blood pressure after two weeks of taking a regular dose of Tylenol.

Patient: I heard it causes liver problems. Is that correct?

Me: Yes, that is a definite side effect when too much Tylenol is ingested. Liver damage can result. Tylenol is the leading cause of acute liver failure in the United States. Each year its active ingredient, acetaminophen, accounts for more than 100,000 poison center calls and 60,000 emergency room visits.

Acetaminophen is the most common drug ingredient in the US. Therefore, it's important to check the labels of other drugs for acetaminophen, including prescription drugs, because there is a chance it is included. More than 600 prescription and over-the-counter drugs have the active ingredient from Tylenol, acetaminophen, in them, so it can be very easy to go over the recommended ceiling of 4000 mg for adults, and 3000 mg for elderly patients.

In addition, combining drugs with alcohol is never a good idea, but because people are often told Tylenol is safe, it may not be thought of as a problem to take it with alcohol. Dr. Joel Weinstock, professor and chief of the Division of Gastroenterology and Hepatology at Tufts New England Medical Center in Boston, told *ABC News* that combining Tylenol with alcohol is very dangerous, and can result in liver failure, and if the patient makes it that long, could require a liver transplant.

Remember, Tylenol's pain-relieving quality is not addressing the problem of where the pain is coming from. Could short-term use be safe if you combine that with trying to find the root cause of the problem? Maybe. But if it is masking the pain, then this can make it very difficult to find and address the root cause of the problem. As discussed in Chapter 1, pain is trying to tell you that something is amiss. If we cover up the pain completely, we have less of a chance to find and correct the underlying problem.

Side Effects of Tylenol

Some side effects can be serious. If you experience any of the following symptoms, stop taking acetaminophen and call your doctor immediately or get emergency medical attention:

- Red, peeling, or blistering skin
- Rash
- Hives
- Itching
- Swelling of the face, throat, tongue, lips, eyes, hands, feet, ankles, or lower legs
- Hoarseness
- Difficulty breathing or swallowing

Oftentimes, when anti-inflammatories or Tylenol don't work and pain persists, doctors may prescribe opioids or nerve pain medications to address the pain. As a matter of fact, at least in my experience, opioids and nerve pain medications are regularly prescribed and considered a standing order to manage pain after surgery. More on that in the next chapter.

Pain Pills for Chronic Muscle and Joint Pain

OPIOIDS

These days, there isn't a lot of education that I have to do for patients regarding opioids. The vast majority of people know opioids are effective for pain relief, but they are also aware of their addictive nature. The opioid epidemic is shared frequently on all news channels, and the movies released about it depict the rise of opioid prescriptions as potentially due to certain pharmaceutical companies putting profits ahead of patient safety, as well as pushing for off-label prescriptions.

An off-label prescription is when a drug is prescribed for a reason outside of its intended use. The intended use has been proven safe and effective, but off-label use is prescribed at the physician's discretion if its benefits appear to outweigh the risks.

Approved drugs have to go through rigorous testing and FDA approval for use in specific circumstances, but as the preceding paragraph points out, the off-label use of medications bypasses that requirement. I have always found the acceptance of off-label somewhat paradoxical since herbs that have been used traditionally for thousands of years are often scrutinized as unsafe, even if there is research to support their use, but off-label use of medications that are not yet approved for uses they are prescribed for aren't looked at with the same critical lens.

According to AHRQ.gov, other reviews report that up to one-third of the scripts written are for off-label use. That's millions of prescriptions for medications that haven't been approved for uses they are being prescribed for, especially when you consider that over 6 billion prescriptions were written in 2022 according to statistics.com.

Often, the patients I see avoid the use of opioids or want to get off opioids as soon as possible. But there are many patients who are using these potent painkillers frequently for pain control, including elderly patients. Despite the research that they are often just as effective as non-opioids for acute pain, and that long-term use of opioids for chronic pain can actually increase sensitivity to pain, they are still being prescribed. People don't realize these meds make you feel more pain when they wear off, which makes opioids very difficult to stop once a person is on them for a while.

Occasionally, people will ask me why their doctor prescribed them an opioid to help with pain resulting from inflammation.

My response is always to discuss this with their prescribing physician, as opioids in some cases, such as palliative cancer care, can be very effective, and I go on to explain that opioids act on different receptors in the body and brain and can be strong anti-inflammatory medications as well as being able to block pain receptors. But are their benefits worth the risk?

How Do Opioids Work?

Think of the constant chronic pain you are experiencing as noise continually being blared in a small room. Because the pain/noise is constantly grabbing your attention, you can't concentrate on what you want to do or think about other than the noise. Now, think of the opioid as noise-cancelling earphones, muffling or blocking out the noise. Add in a touch of euphoria from opioids' effects on the reward systems in the brain, and the person not only doesn't hear the noise (feel the pain), but they feel on top of the world . . . that is, until the opioid wears off. Then, the pain can often be worse than what was previously felt, a phenomenon called hyperalgesia. This is one of the reasons these pain medications can be highly addictive. Tolerance also becomes an issue. People tend to need to take more to achieve the same euphoric state and pain relief that the previously lower dose provided. This can eventually lead to overdose and death.

Center for Disease Control's List of Common Opioids and Side Effects:

- Methadone
- Oxycodone (such as OxyContin®)
- Hydrocodone (such as Vicodin®)

Side Effects of Opioids:

- Tolerance—meaning you might need to keep taking more of the medication for the same pain relief
- Physical dependence—meaning you have symptoms of withdrawal when the medication is stopped
- Increased sensitivity to pain
- Constipation
- Nausea, vomiting, and dry mouth
- Sleepiness and dizziness
- Confusion
- Depression
- Low levels of testosterone that can result in lower sex drive, energy, and strength
- Itching and sweating

When NSAIDs Don't Work and You Don't Want Opioids

ENTER GABAPENTIN

When anti-inflammatories don't work, or the patient doesn't want to go on opioids, or opioids are not indicated, a recent medication that has been prescribed more often is called Gabapentin. Gabapentin's approved use at the time of this writing is for epilepsy, post-herpetic neuralgia, and restless leg syndrome. But its off-label use for nerve pain appears to be increasing and will likely be approved by the FDA at some point for this purpose, if not already by the time of publication. Scientists and medical professionals don't know exactly how it works, but they believe it affects GABA receptors in the body in some way. It targets the GABA receptors and there is evidence that GABA helps to slow down and inhibit neurotransmitters in the brain that help create and maintain a state of calm.

A forty-year-old patient of mine named Michelle came to the clinic with chronic back and leg discomfort. Prior to seeing me, she went to her physician several times to figure out why she wasn't getting relief. She had injured her back months prior, and the leg discomfort did not subside. Her toes started to become numb, and her foot began to feel weaker, too. She wanted to know if her doctor would recommend surgery. He and another physician that she saw for a second opinion both said that, based on her MRI, they wouldn't recommend surgery. They did prescribe her a drug called Gabapentin that helped with the intensity of the symptoms but did not get rid of them completely. She had no idea it was not approved for leg and foot numbness at that time, but she thought it was helping her because when she tried to decrease it, the symptoms would come back.

She was also unaware of the risks associated with taking this medication longer term, such as the potential for psychological and physical dependence.

How Does Gabapentin Work?

Although scientists and medical doctors really don't know how Gabapentin works for nerve pain, we can liken it to the music analogy related to opioids. Gabapentin's mechanism of action can be understood using that same room filled with annoying music (the pain) that refuses to allow you to concentrate, or even get a restful sleep. Imagine the speaker that this music is playing from has the old school wires (nervous system) connecting it to its source or console (brain).

Gabapentin acts like a volume knob on the stereo (brain) that can turn down the intensity of the music. It doesn't switch off flow through the wires (nervous system) entirely, but it reduces the volume, making the noise (pain/discomfort) more bearable or low enough that it isn't noticeable.

When Gabapentin is taken, it works to turn down the volume by inhibiting specific signals in the nervous system. The noise is still there as stated, but it's less intense, reducing the pain and discomfort.

Pain signals, like electrical signals along the speaker wire, are transmitted through nerve pathways. Therefore, in essence, Gabapentin doesn't stop the 'music' of pain entirely, instead, it reduces its 'volume' to a more manageable level, offering relief but not stopping the reason why the music (pain) is blaring.

This was exactly what was happening with Michelle. She still couldn't exercise due to the pain and weakness she was experiencing, but she could function and sleep if she took the Gabapentin throughout the day and evening to turn down the intensity of the pain. Unfortunately, without being able to exercise, she gained weight and was feeling very frustrated, and that is when she came to my clinic.

Common Side Effects of Gabapentin

Common side effects of Gabapentin include:

- Feeling tired
- Dizziness
- Headache
- Nausea and vomiting
- Fever
- Difficulty speaking
- Recurring infections
- Memory loss
- Weight gain
- Movement problems: coordination problems, being unsteady, tremors, jerky movements
- Unusual eye movements, double vision
- Breathing difficulties

More serious side effects related to use of Gabapentin are:

- Kidney toxicity if there are already problems with the kidney
- Serious breathing problems when used with CNS depressants, as well as patients with lung problems
- Symptoms of withdrawal and dependence when Gabapentin is stopped can include nausea, dizziness, headaches, insomnia, and anxiety

Is Gabapentin the Next Overuse Epidemic?

According to the *Journal of the American Medical Association Network* published in July of 2022, between the years 2019-2020, Gabapentin was detected in almost 10 percent of the nearly 60,000 overdose deaths during that time, and Gabapentin was determined to be the actual cause of death in approximately 3,000 of those cases.

Muscle Relaxants: An Old Option Coming Back in Style

While helping people with joint and muscle pain for over three decades, I have witnessed many trends. Muscle relaxants, in my experience, are prescribed less often in chronic pain, and most often for shorter periods, also due to their addictive nature. But lately, I have been noticing a trend of muscle relaxants coming back onto the scene.

How Do Muscle Relaxants Work?

Picture a garden surrounded by a gate that's locked tight, representing muscles that are tense and in spasm after an injury. Remember from Chapter 2, the body wants to protect you from creating further damage after an injury so the muscles around the injured part can go into lockdown mode, preventing further movement as the first responders are called to the area of injury to get to work initiating the healing process.

Muscle relaxants act like a key that unlocks the gate. When the key turns, the gate opens, and the tension in the muscles can ease, even if the injury still needs time to heal.

But because muscle relaxants are most frequently given to the patient to be taken by mouth, this 'unlocking' effect can affect the whole body systemically, which results in the patient not being able to function normally. Patients are cautioned not to drive a car or operate machinery while taking these medications.

Steve, who we talked about in the last chapter, took muscle relaxants for a while for his low back pain, but had to stop as he found he couldn't function at work when he took them. He would experience a hangover feeling after taking them the night before to help him sleep. And he often felt irritated or nervous the day after.

A large review of many research articles determined that muscle relaxants and NSAIDs may reduce pain for acute back injuries better than placebos, whereas acetaminophen (Tylenol) did not. But the benefits of muscle relaxants for chronic low back pain did not show a clear effect. Despite this, the prescriptions for muscle relaxants tripled between 2005-2016.

It's typically recommended that they not be used for longer than three weeks, as they have been shown to be ineffective beyond this time. But patients of mine have come to me after being on them for four or more weeks for persistent back pain, which is the relaxants' most common use.

Muscle relaxants tend to pose a bigger risk to elderly patients, and the American Geriatrics Society recommends they not be used in that population. Yet one study reported that 22 percent of office visits where muscle relaxants were prescribed were for seniors, and when you consider that seniors make up 14 percent of the population, that amount of prescribing is significant.

The study was based on national prescribing data from 2005 to 2016. The researchers looked at the total number of visits per year, which medications were prescribed, and if the prescription was new or ongoing.

Dr. Charles Leonard, assistant professor of epidemiology at

Pennsylvania State University, said the research did not look specifically at why doctors were prescribing these medications more, but he suspects there are at least a few factors driving the increase. One is that there aren't really any good alternative drugs, so doctors may not want to take them away. Another is that patients may put some pressure on their doctor to treat their pain and with the decrease in opioid prescriptions, muscle relaxants seem to be making a comeback.

And though muscle relaxants tend to perform slightly better than placebos in the general population, they show no significant benefit over utilizing NSAIDs or even physical therapy for pain relief.

Cleveland Clinic List of Common Muscle Relaxants and Side Effects

- Carisoprodol (Soma®, Vanadom®)
- Chlorzoxazone (Lorzone®, Parafon Forte DSC®, Relax-DS®, Remular S®)
- Cyclobenzaprine (Fexmid®, Flexeril®)
- Methocarbamol (Robaxin®)
- Baclofen (Lioresal®)
- Dantrolene (Dantrium®)
- Tizanidine (Zanaflex®)
- Diazepam (Valium®)

Side effects:

- Drowsiness and fatigue
- Dizziness
- Nausea
- Headache
- Dry mouth
- Fainting
- Blurred vision

Polypharmacy Common for Pain Control

Polypharmacy for pain refers to the use of multiple medications simultaneously to manage pain, often in patients with chronic or complex conditions. This approach is common in cases where a single drug is insufficient to control pain, and multiple drugs targeting different mechanisms are attempted to reduce the pain so a patient can function. While polypharmacy can be effective in improving pain management, it also carries risks, particularly related to drug interactions, side effects, and patient safety.

A friend of mine, Liz, was prescribed Gabapentin, carbamazepine (another drug used in epilepsy), and NSAIDs for her severe pain from trigeminal neuralgia. The trigeminal nerve in the face is also responsible for biting and chewing. This condition is often called 'the suicide pain' because for many people, it does not go away, and makes normal functions like eating, talking, and washing very difficult. The only recommendations for treatment are medication and surgery.

Fortunately, Liz did a lot of her own research. After four hellish months of constant pain every few hours, all day and night when the meds wore off, Liz decided to try lifting her head much higher to sleep. She used two pillows, and within a week, her pain went away. Liz was fortunate that her side effects from withdrawing from Gabapentin were mild.

A Cocktail of Drugs Following Surgery

When I heard my friend was struggling after her total joint replacement, I knew I had to see her. I've seen hundreds of patients after surgery, so I expected to find her in pain, and maybe a bit down, but I wasn't prepared for what I walked into. The room was quiet, almost too quiet, and there she was, buried under a floral comforter that seemed to swallow her whole. Her eyes, glassy and distant, fluttered as she fought to stay awake, her chin dipping toward her chest with each question I asked her. I could sense that something wasn't right, and I knew I had to stay a little longer—something in the air told me this visit was going to be more than just a quick check-in.

"I am taking Julie to soccer practice," my friend's husband said, as he set the white paper plate with the browned grilled cheese by her side.

She slowly turned her head and looked up at him, replying, "Thanks."

He looked at me and then at her. I smiled, and he shrugged his shoulders and turned to head toward the garage. I decided to stay, at least until she fell asleep, so she did not feel alone. But to my pleasant surprise, after a few bites of the sandwich, she began to perk up a little.

"Oh my gosh, that's the best grilled cheese sandwich I've had in my life!" She smiled, and I laughed as she took another bite.

"How are you feeling?" I asked as I pulled my chair closer to the side of her bed where her surgical knee hid under the comforter.

"I am exhausted, and I feel nauseous all the time," she said, setting her paper plate at her side as her sandwich slid halfway off, teetering on touching the bed sheets. She sat up a little. "The doctors told me to stay ahead of the pain, so I have to wake up every few hours during the night to take my meds."

"What?" I asked. "You should be getting some sleep. Sleep is going to help with the healing process," I insisted.

"I know, that's what I am thinking too." She wiped her forehead. "Ugh, I have to get up and go to the bathroom."

"What are you taking?" I asked as I stood up, contemplating whether I should help her.

"Oxy, some anti-inflammatories, and gaba something or other." She responded as she removed the comforter and slowly swung her surgical leg over the side of the bed.

"Gabapentin?" I queried.

"Yeah, that's the one," she replied as she stood up.

"Wow, that's quite the cocktail," I commented as I positioned myself to assist in case she lost her balance. *Polypharmacy at work again.*

As she stood and paused to adjust her crutches, I could observe her bandaged knee. It was swollen so much that her kneecap wasn't visible, and a covering was placed over the incision that was full of dried blood. It extended from above her kneecap to a couple of inches below. "Look out. I have to use the bathroom."

I moved out of her way. "Let me know if you need some help."

"I am just happy you are here, in case I fall or something," she replied, and her face winced a bit as she slowly lowered her heel to the floor.

As she hobbled off to the bathroom, I asked, "Are you sure that is what they said? About staying ahead of the pain?"

"Yep, pretty sure," she said from inside the bathroom.

I wasn't too concerned about her falling. I knew she would have had plenty of instruction from her physical therapists in the hospital. And despite being cautious, she looked quite steady with her crutches.

I was, however, concerned that she was told to take her pain meds "to get ahead of the pain," and was convinced this was either a misunderstanding or just that particular hospital's policy. That is until a year and a half later, 400 miles away, as I sat in the post-op recovery room with my twenty-one-year-old son when he was given his prescription medications following his ACL surgery repair after an injury playing college football.

A Common Practice

The hard paper bag crinkled, and the medications shook slightly as the nurse handed his prescription medications to my son as he was propped up in his postoperative bed. She was very pleasant and thorough during his surgery prep and was very kind to me while I waited for him to return to his room after the reconstructive knee surgery. I noticed the package she handed him included a few white pieces of paper with postoperative instructions.

"So here are your medications: oxycodone, Gabapentin, and NSAIDs. Make sure you take them every six hours to stay ahead of the pain."

I felt my jaw drop and my eyes widen. *Oh, hell no, she did not just say that!*

My son's pale face and sunken eyes looked at me and then back at the nurse. This was my cue to take the meds and the papers from her. I stood up and forced a smile as she handed me the white paper bags.

As I sat back down, I waited for her to explain to him, a twenty-one-year-old young man, about the dangers related to opioid medications and what to do to make sure he did not become reliant on them.

Those instructions never came.

"Any questions?" she asked.

My son looked at me with his dilated pupils and dry, chapped lips. Despite the remainder of anesthesia still coursing through his system, he knew that I would have questions.

"So, you want him to wake up if he is resting, to take all of these medications?"

"If he wants to stay ahead of the pain."

I was sure I did not hear her right. I sat up a little taller, scooted to the edge of my chair and leaned in.

"But what about the rest that he needs?"

At this point, my son straightened up in his recovery bed as if the adrenaline of potential embarrassment started to sober him up. His slightly dazed gaze turned abruptly into a stink eye that translated into the familiar 'seriously Mom, don't embarrass me' look that I had definitely seen plenty of times before. I tried not to look at him, but I felt his stare piercing through my attempts to ignore his response. My posture relaxed and as I slid to the back of my chair, I felt the cool vinyl covering the seat on the back of my pant legs contrast with the heat of irritation building up from my neck to the top of my head.

The nurse stood with one hand on each end of the stethoscope around her neck and inquired, "Did you want to ask something?"

Taking a deep breath, I crossed my legs and set my hands on top of the pill bottles in the paper bag. The noise of the paper crinkling accompanied by a slight rattle of the bottle broke the silence first, as I exhaled and then responded. "Nope, all good. Thanks."

I kept smiling at them both through the frustration, thinking about the statistics related to opioid overuse and addiction. According to Harvard University, a purported 7 percent of opioid-naive patients, patients who never had taken an opioid before, can be at risk for overuse. And if that doesn't seem like a lot, think about the fact that there are over 50 million surgeries performed per year.

The data is lacking as to whether or not giving these medications contributes to decreasing the development of chronic pain. But as discussed, there IS data to support medications such as opioids contributing to hyperalgesia, i.e., an increased sensitivity to feeling pain and an extreme response to pain.

There was also no discussion about the side effects of the NSAIDs or Gabapentin. All this information was indeed on the discharge papers, but a quick review of the information would have been a great service to my son because, at twenty-one, he wasn't likely to read any of it without encouragement from someone other than his mom.

I let him be the judge of what he needed for the long, four-hour car ride home. He did not take the cocktail recommended to 'stay ahead of the pain.' One NSAID sufficed. And when he arrived home, he applied the RICE method (rested, iced, kept his knee compression bandage on, and elevated his knee), and slept soundly through the next few nights. His young healthy body was able to help him gradually resolve the inflammation and make it through his acute phase of pain.

These two scenarios related to the cocktail of medications often routinely prescribed after surgery once again opened my eyes to the generally accepted (over)use of medications that:

1. Could be addictive
2. May be unnecessary
3. Could contribute to the development of long-term issues related to pain

Nowhere on the sheets that were handed to my son was there any information about how he could control the pain and inflammation without the assistance of these potentially unnecessary and addictive medications.

And please remember, I am not against taking all medications. I am against the use of medications unnecessarily, and the lack of education about how to address pain and inflammation without reliance on medications so that patients have a choice in how they want to direct their care. I grew up with pain medications and even anti-inflammatory meds being nonexistent in our house, or at the very least a last resort, versus a seemingly required first-line treatment. It's my hope that those who want to go back to the traditional approach to medications as a last resort (unless a life-threatening scenario exists) will have information to help them achieve the knowledge necessary to make this happen, and still live an active lifestyle where pain does not limit their ability to participate fully in the things they want to do.

Additional Injections Gaining More Traction for Joint Pain

Patients often ask me about injections considered as an alternative to other medical treatments. I don't administer these treatments in my clinic, as we provide cost-effective alternatives that are noninvasive, but I wanted to mention them here to help you understand what they are and how they are used in case you want to discuss them with your provider. Research is growing as science begins to underpin their use.

Alternative Invasive Means of Joint Pain Relief

While I strongly advise my patients to avoid getting cortisone injections if at all possible due to the new research about the long-term negative effects that have been associated with using them, there are other types of injections that are being used to help with joint pain, both acute and chronic, that do not have the negative side effects of cortisone. Examples of these are platelet rich plasma injections (PRP), platelet rich fibrin (PRF) injections, gel shots or hyaluronic acid injections, and stem cell injections.

One of the upsides of these shots is that when given by competent providers, there do not seem to be any negative side effects associated with having them, beyond the side effects of receiving any injections. And there is research, with varied outcomes, that in some cases can support their use in certain people with mild to moderate arthritic changes in their joints.

But the downside is that they are expensive, ranging anywhere from $1,000 each up to $10,000 or more. And simply because they are injections, this poses a downside to those who would rather have a noninvasive treatment.

The idea behind these treatments is to stimulate the body's own healing process with either autologous cells (cells from our own body) in PRP, PRF, and stem cell injections, or substances similar to what is already in our body, i.e., the gel/hyaluronic acid shots, a substance that is, according to the Mayo Clinic, "similar to a substance that occurs naturally in the joints." That substance acts as a lubricant and a shock absorber.

PRP Injections

Platelet-rich plasma (PRP) injections are a treatment used for various conditions, including chronic joint and muscle pain. This therapy involves extracting a small amount of the patient's blood, processing it to concentrate the platelets, and then re-injecting this platelet-rich plasma into the affected area. Platelets are known for their role in healing and regeneration. They release growth factors that increase the recruitment of cells that can promote tissue repair. In the context of inflammation and chronic pain in joints or muscles, PRP aims to initiate and accelerate the body's natural healing process. It is often used for conditions like tendinitis, arthritis, and muscle injuries, where traditional treatments haven't been effective.

One meta-analysis showed that PRP injections were effective in relieving pain from knee osteoarthritis, ankle osteoarthritis, and TMJ osteoarthritis, but not hip osteoarthritis.

PRF Injections

Platelet-rich fibrin (PRF) injections offer a promising alternative treatment for joint issues, leveraging the body's natural healing mechanisms. Unlike other platelet therapies, PRF contains a higher concentration of growth factors and cytokines, which are crucial for tissue repair and regeneration. The fibrin matrix in PRF acts as a scaffold, gradually releasing these growth factors to the affected area, enhancing cell proliferation and accelerating healing.

One of the key advantages of PRF is its natural origin; like PRP, it is derived from the patient's own blood, significantly reducing the risk of immune reactions or complications. Furthermore, PRF injections have been shown to improve joint pain, reduce inflammation, and enhance joint function in conditions like osteoarthritis. Studies suggest that PRF can stimulate cartilage regeneration and reduce the progression of joint degeneration, making it a valuable option for those seeking to delay or avoid surgical interventions.

A research study with three-year follow-up showed that PRP injections combined with PRF yielded better results than PRP alone.

Compared to corticosteroid injections, which provide temporary relief but can lead to joint deterioration over time, PRF promotes long-term healing and tissue repair without the adverse side effects. This makes PRF a particularly attractive option for individuals looking for a more sustainable and natural approach to managing joint pain and improving joint health.

Combination therapy does seem to be emerging in the research as the best approach. Shockwave therapy that you will learn about in Chapter 7 has also been shown to enhance the effects of these injections.

Gel Shots: The Body's Natural Lubricant

Gel shots and hyaluronic acid injections are often used interchangeably as they both refer to viscosupplementation, a treatment primarily used for knee osteoarthritis. Hyaluronic acid is a naturally occurring substance in the joint fluid that acts as a lubricant and shock absorber. In osteoarthritis, the quality and quantity of hyaluronic acid diminish, leading to increased joint pain and stiffness. By injecting hyaluronic acid directly into the joint, these gel shots aim to restore the normal balance, reduce pain, and improve mobility. They are particularly beneficial for patients who have not found relief from other treatments like physical therapy or NSAIDs. Although primarily used for knee arthritis, these injections can also be applied to other joints.

Research has shown that hyaluronic acid shots tend not to be harmful, but their efficacy in treating osteoarthritic joints can be hit or miss. PRP injections tend to fare better in some studies that compare the two injections head-to-head.

Stem Cell Injections

Stem cell injections are an emerging treatment in the field of regenerative medicine, used for addressing chronic pain and inflammation in joints and muscles. These injections involve using stem cells, which have the unique ability to develop into different types of cells to promote the healing of damaged tissues. The stem cells can be harvested from the patient's bone marrow, fat tissue, or blood. Once collected, they are processed and then injected into the affected area or given intravenously. The theory behind stem cell therapy is that these cells can help in repairing damaged tissue, reducing inflammation, and ultimately alleviating pain. This treatment is considered for a variety of conditions, including osteoarthritis, tendon injuries, and muscle strains. However, it's important to note that stem cell therapy is still a relatively new approach, and more research is needed to fully understand its efficacy and long-term outcomes.

A review of the literature showed that stem cell therapy has promise, but researchers found it difficult to compare studies due to different sources of the stem cells used, as well as varying doses. This inconsistency in treatment appears to affect the outcomes. Once consensus is reached and outcomes become more consistent, stem cell injections may be deemed an effective treatment for osteoarthritis.

PRP, PRF, stem cell and hyaluronic acid injections do show promise, but when combined with shockwave therapy (which you will learn about in Part 2), the results are much better than any of these injections used on their own.

Serious Questions Remain

There is clear evidence that the medications both synthetic and natural (autologous, coming from our own body) discussed in this chapter can be effective at reducing pain or inflammation and make patients more comfortable after injury. But serious questions remain about prescription or over-the-counter medications continued use after initial prescription due to the possible long-term side effects (such as hyperalgesia, i.e., increased pain sensitivity), especially for opioids and other medications that have potential for abuse.

Science does show that some medications mentioned in this chapter disrupt the body's natural healing response to an acute injury or a chronic issue such as arthritis. These medications can clearly have deleterious effects on your overall health, including joints, muscles, and other systems of the body, especially when taken ong-term.

Using these medications has become an easy fix when many providers stuck in a broken health system are forced to average ten minutes or less with each patient, and when patients demand quick options for relief with their evidence coming from the latest advertisement. Based on patients that I speak with every day, I am convinced that if given a choice of becoming dependent on any of these medications or seeking an effective alternative, they would choose a noninvasive or perhaps less invasive approach if they are provided with all of the information about the consequences attached to quick fixes.

As discussed, especially with chronic conditions, these medications are not addressing the underlying cause of the pain, and though they allow short-term relief after acute trauma like surgery or significant injury, relying on these medications in the long-term and, one could argue, even in the short-term, is similar to what *Chicken Soup for The Soul* and *The Success Principles* author Jack Canfield once told me.

Canfield likens using these medications to tune out the pain signals to taking the batteries out of a smoke alarm in your house when it is blaring because of a fire. Whatever caused the alarm to go off is not going to go away when you take the batteries out. The fire keeps smoldering whether you can hear the alarm or not.

In other words, none of these medications are able to remove the true underlying cause of the inflammation and subsequently the pain and heightened sensitivity that is causing you to have chronic pain in the first place. And in the worst-case scenario, some of these medications may not only make your pain worse in the long run, but they can also have deleterious effects on other important organ systems of your body such as the liver and kidneys. In addition, the potential for addiction when prescriptions for medications such as opioids are not monitored and not ceased after a short time is real.

NOTE: Please remember that I am not opposed to medications. I am opposed to the overuse of medications and not looking for long-term solutions to avoid medication if possible. I help patients work around medications that they may rely on whenever possible, as well. But many people have no idea there are few long-term studies to determine the effects of medications that at first were prescribed for short-term treatment but then are continued for years, even decades after. There are many ways to manage chronic pain or pain after surgery to help assist in the patient's healing process. Medications may play a part in that, but the advice to wake up in the middle of a restful sleep to take medication to "stay ahead of the pain" does not make sense to me.

Do I want patients to be in debilitating pain? No, of course not. But I also want patients to be educated about how their body can help them heal and what they can do to improve their pain levels that doesn't involve the continuous consumption of potentially addictive narcotics. There is a balance that can be achieved.

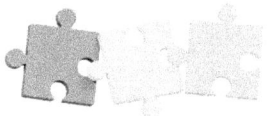

Key Pieces

Inflammation's Role: Inflammation is not inherently bad; it's a natural and necessary response to injury. While conventional treatments focus on suppressing inflammation with medications like NSAIDs, this can interfere with the body's natural healing process and potentially lead to chronic pain.

Limitations of NSAIDs and Other Medications: NSAIDs and other medications described as anti-inflammatories, while useful for short-term pain relief, may prevent proper healing if overused. They can reduce the body's natural response to inflammation, which can result in long-term complications and a higher risk of developing chronic pain.

Risks of Steroid Injections: Cortisone and other steroid injections, while effective in the short term, can have significant long-term side effects, including accelerated joint deterioration, increased risk of tendon tears, and rarely, potential cardiovascular risks.

Caution with Pain Medications: Medications like opioids and Gabapentin are often prescribed to manage pain, but they come with risks, including dependence, increased sensitivity to pain, and other side effects. These medications may have their place, but they do not address the root cause of pain and can complicate the healing process.

Exploring Alternative Injections: Newer treatments like PRP, hyaluronic acid, and stem cell injections offer alternatives to conventional pain management. While these treatments show promise, they can be costly, and outcomes may vary. Combining these with other therapies, like shockwave therapy, may yield better results.

CHAPTER 4

Surgical Shadows
Understanding the Risks and Limitations of Going Under the Knife

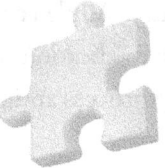

"Caution, not excess, is the principal of the wise."

–Author unknown

It was the end of the summer as I sat in the waiting room on the hard, cold, plastic seats, wondering when my name would be called. I glanced over at the CDs I had next to me that had the results of my X-ray and MRI of my knee. I thought about what I saw on the test results and their reports and felt confident that after treating patients with this type of injury before, I knew what structures were likely responsible for the loud audible pop and searing ice pick-like pain that I experienced on the inside of my knee while teaching my son how to do the polka at a family wedding. But I wanted to consult with a colleague to see if they had any other input.

I sighed as I looked at my phone and realized I had been waiting for thirty minutes already. First, they took an X-ray of my knee. I was told the one I had already brought in may not be sufficient, so they wanted to do their own. I tried to ignore the thoughts about excess costs related to our healthcare system because I just wanted to go with the flow.

You are a patient here, Stacey, I said to myself. *You aren't here as a healthcare provider.*

I resisted the urge to check my phone again and instead found myself chuckling at the memory of dragging my leg behind me after my injury like some old skit in the movie *Young Frankenstein*. *Man, how I wish there was a video of me trying to get back to my car.* I was brought back to the present after hearing my name called in the distance. I looked up at the medical assistant (MA) holding the heavy wooden door open while waiting for me to walk through it.

She stayed behind me, and I heard her over my shoulder instructing me to go into the third room on the left. Another large wooden door clicked closed as I sat down in a new cold, hard, plastic chair. The MA reviewed my past medical history and asked about medications, supplements, and everything they needed for my medical record. I watched her as she tapped away on the keyboard, opened my mouth obligingly as she took my temperature and offered my sleeveless arm for the blood pressure cuff. Her voice was slightly muffled as she spoke through her light blue mask.

After a bit more chit-chat, she said the doctor would be with me shortly. As she left the room, she switched on the computer monitor that showed the X-ray of my knee on the screen.

I get strangely excited to see these types of results. Call me crazy, but the human body is so very interesting to me. My chair screeched over the floor as I pulled it closer to the monitor on the desk.

I took my readers from the top of my head and set them on the bridge of my nose to see the black-and-white images on the computer monitor. I leaned in to take a look. *Hmm, much better than the old days of large plastic sheets stuck up on a lighted background for the doctor to review.* I could see the forty-year-old screws that looked like they were floating in my knee after they were drilled into the bone to reattach my new ACL back in 1986. Just then, the latch of the door clicked, and the doctor in the traditional white coat with blue scrubs and the obligatory stethoscope dangling around her neck walked in.

My Life-Changing Moment

The doctor introduced herself. I was happy to see a female as an orthopedic surgeon. They are usually men, so this was a pleasant surprise. I was hopeful that as two female health professionals, we would connect.

My hopes of building any professional rapport were put on hold as she got right down to business, asking questions about what had happened. During this time, her eyes darted from the details on the other computer screen to the clear clipboard that held the sheet of paper I filled out as I checked in at the front desk. The quick pace of the appointment shouldn't have surprised me, as physicians typically only have roughly ten minutes with each patient to keep on schedule.

After exchanging pleasantries and asking how I felt, the doctor stood up and motioned to the padded table next to us. That, I assumed, meant hop up on the table for an examination. I grabbed the desk in front of me and took a step toward the exam table. Just then, a shot of pain ran down the inside of my knee toward my calf. I hesitated, closed my eyes, took a breath in quickly, then slowly let it out as the pain faded away. After I opened my eyes, the doctor replied, "Looks like it hurts pretty bad."

"Yes, it does," I replied as I hobbled over and placed my injured leg on the step next to the table and both butt cheeks eventually plopped on the edge, scrunching the thin white paper covering the vinyl.

I watched her as she looked at my knee. I could feel my muscles let go with hesitation like the rachets on a wrench. They were still trying their best to protect me. She pressed on the swollen areas on my bent knee silently and my arms tensed. She pulled out the metal extension at the end of the table that sounded like opening a metal file cabinet.

"You can relax and lie back," she said, gesturing to the head of the table.

At least it's not the gynecologist, I thought as I lay back. After heaving both feet up on the metal extension plate, the doctor started to move my knee to check for ligament or meniscus damage. I immediately regretted not shaving my legs. My patients always apologized for that to me during an exam, but now it was me with the embarrassing bristles.

The whole exam took about two minutes, which was a bit disappointing, but not unusual. The clock was ticking. From the chest pocket of her white lab coat, she pulled out a pen and walked back to her chair to sit down. She gestured to my empty chair and I followed her lead, hopping off onto my uninjured leg and then gingerly placing the affected leg on the ground. I tensed my whole body for a moment and then felt my muscles release. *Good*, I thought as I managed to get back to my seat, *no stabbing pain*.

We now sat face-to-face, with the computer monitors off to the side in between us. My X-rays were in my peripheral vision, and I was excited that soon, I was sure, she would begin to reference them and show me what she thought happened to my knee. I rustled in my seat anxiously waiting to see if she agreed with my hypothesis. I was curious if she thought it was the medial collateral ligament, the medial meniscus, or scar tissue that had built up from my surgery almost forty years prior that had created the pop and pain. I couldn't wait to tell her my opinion, and then we would discuss it like colleagues and come up with a plan.

"Well, looking at your X-ray, I can see a significant amount of arthritis," she raised her pen to the X-ray displayed on the monitor. The point of her pen moved across several areas that, sure enough, looked bumpy and uneven, definitely resembling arthritis. I could clearly see what she was referring to, and if it weren't for the identifiable screws, for a moment, I thought she may have had the wrong X-ray. I would have assumed with that much arthritis that I should have had pain long before the pop.

She continued. "Really, you have only two options: a total knee replacement or an injection to stave off the pain until you are ready for the total knee replacement."

I shook my head trying to rewind the conversation because I was sure I had heard her incorrectly.

"A total knee replacement?" I parroted. "But I did not have any pain before I heard the pop."

"Yes, but you can clearly see, here, and here, and here, that your knee is full of arthritis. There's no cure for that except a total knee replacement."

"But those places you pointed aren't where my pain is," I responded.

She sat quietly and looked annoyed for a moment. At this point, she hadn't enquired about my occupation.

I tried to keep my voice in a normal tone, disguising my building frustration. "Based on my MRI report that you have, the X-ray you did, and your exam, what do you think the pop was? A ligament, the meniscus, scar tissue, or what?"

"Well, your ligaments felt intact on the exam, and the MRI report shows tears in both meniscus and a sprained ligament. But it really doesn't matter what the pop was, the film shows your knee is a mess."

I felt heat rising up from my neck to my ears. I took a deep breath and continued, "Okay. I see what you are talking about," I said as I gestured to the X-ray, "but clearly the arthritis was there way before the incident at the wedding, and my knee wasn't hurting before the pop," I repeated. "The arthritis and even the torn meniscus on both sides did not happen in that one instance. So why would I want to have a major operation like a total knee replacement if the arthritis isn't and wasn't causing me any pain previous to this incident?"

"Look," she responded as she laid her pen and her clipboard on the small table where the computer monitor sat. Folding her hands in her lap, she continued, "I see patients with this type of arthritis every day, and they put off the procedure as long as they can until it's so bad they can't stand it anymore, and then they come back for the surgery."

She did not seem to hear a word I said. I took another deep breath and asked her about any alternatives, such as an arthroscopic surgery to investigate if there were any fragments floating around inside the knee. Maybe a bone spur broke off or something?

Her reply was, "Research doesn't support doing a clean-out like that anymore."

Fair enough, I thought. I had read the same research.

"If I am going in that knee," she said, as she pointed toward the display with her pen, "I am doing a replacement."

"What about stem cell injections or hyaluronic acid injections?"

"Those are possible, but they are expensive. We don't do them, and they are not covered by insurance. The research is still not conclusive about them. And in a knee like yours..."

I felt my eyeballs wanting to roll, but I resisted.

"I wouldn't recommend any of those options." She paused, then continued. "The only other thing I can offer you today is a cortisone injection."

She looked at her watch, and I took a quick glance at my phone. Twelve minutes had passed.

"No thanks," I said.

"Do you mind if I ask why not," she inquired.

I really was trying to be a patient and not a healthcare professional with decades of experience. *But what the heck*, I thought. *She asked.*

"Well, research shows," and with those few words, she lifted her pen from the clipboard and looked at the bottom of the sheet I filled in where I listed my occupation. She cleared her throat and sat up slightly in her chair as she met my eyes again, "that cortisone injections can accelerate degeneration so," pointing at the X-ray, "with this significant arthritis that you pointed out in my knee, I don't want to inject something that is likely to make it even worse than it is right now."

She waved her hand in the air like she was swatting a fly away from her face, and said, "Oh, you would have to have hundreds of injections of cortisone to have that type of an effect."

It was right then that I knew our conversation was over.

I leaned back slowly in my chair and felt my forehead furrow, took a deep breath while I gathered my thoughts and replied. "I appreciate your opinion, but I guess we will just have to agree to disagree," I said, all the while thinking, *I wonder how many patients she has given that inaccurate information to? This simply encourages them to have the injection despite new evidence that shows the detrimental effects of cortisone.*

"Okay then," the legs of the chair screeched across the tile floor as the orthopedic surgeon got up from her chair, "you can head back out front and give us a call when you need us."

I smiled weakly and thought *fat chance*, then thanked her for her time, knowing full well I was never going to step foot into that office again. I got the feeling she was likely 100 percent fine with that.

The door slowly closed behind her. I got dressed and limped my way down the hallway, where the lovely medical assistant was there to escort me to the exit. I politely thanked her and the receptionist as I walked past the front desk. I pushed through the revolving doors, and the heat of the afternoon in August rushed onto my face as I walked toward my car. I heard the car door unlock as I grabbed the handle to open the driver's side door, and another wave of warm air, this time from inside the car, enveloped my body. Pivoting on my uninjured leg, I spun myself around to maneuver my backside first into the driver's seat.

Finally, after I was nestled behind the steering wheel, I placed the palms of my hands gingerly on the hot wheel and as I gradually wrapped my fingers around it and I wondered:

- How many people were having surgery as the primary intervention after a conversation like that when it should be the last resort?
- How many people thought that their joint pain was coming from arthritis just because arthritis was pointed out in an X-ray

and then have undergone a major operation and still ended up having pain or problems because the actual cause of their pain wasn't being addressed?
- How many people had cortisone injection after cortisone injection that actually set them up for increasing the arthritis in their joints and making surgery nearly inevitable?

Knowing that my knee was full of arthritis actually empowered me to show that doctor and all my patients that just because you have arthritis, that doesn't mean you have to have pain or surgery. Surgery absolutely works and is necessary for many, but not for all. So it was at that point that the *Pain-Free Formula* was born.

Why I Did Not Have Surgery

Since sharing my experience with others, some have asked, "Why did not you just go ahead with the surgery anyway? Maybe you could prevent the knee from getting worse and avoid a lot of pain later."

My response to those enquiring minds has been, "If I don't have pain, and can still work out and do what I want, I don't really care how much arthritis I have in my knee."

And thankfully, by following the principles you will learn in Part Two of this book, I haven't needed knee surgery and remain active working out and participating in an active lifestyle.

Though surgery is truly a good option for some people, especially after a fall or an accident that results in broken bones or severed ligaments or tendons. It certainly can be life-changing in a positive way, but it doesn't work for and is not necessary for everyone.

Unnecessary Procedures

One of my goals of this book is to help you identify if you could be the one who successfully avoids surgery, or if there is a way that you can be sure that surgery is the absolute right choice for you. Because the bottom line is in the United States, an overwhelming number of surgeries are being performed unnecessarily.

- A study from 2014 reported that 44 percent of the 600,000-plus knee replacements done were unnecessary.
- In 2018, the *Journal of the American Medical Association* (*JAMA*) reported that nearly one-third of hip and knee replacements are unnecessary.
- In 2019, Dr. Kevin Stone, an orthopedic surgeon, said that nearly 80 percent of total knee replacements are not necessary. He claimed that there are other options available instead of a total joint replacement, citing that nearly 50 percent of knee replacement surgeries result in pain in the replaced knee up to ten years later.

When Surgery Doesn't Work: The Increasing Rates of Revisions

It was 11:00 a.m. My mom picked up the phone on my second attempt to reach her. She sounded groggy and a little out of it. As she cleared her throat with a raspy, almost unrecognizable voice, she called out, "Hello?"

"Mom? It's me. How are you?"

"Oh, hi!" she answered back. "I'm fine. Just a little sore."

I was sure "a little sore" was an understatement. My mom, a seventy-five-year-old at that time, had just undergone the third revision of her knee replacement. Her first knee replacement just did not feel right, and the surgeon told her to be patient. It could take up to a year to feel normal again. She waited past the year and her knee was still hot to the touch and sore. She broke out in a rash around the knee as well, which eventually began to spread around her entire body. No infection was detected in her system, but there was clearly something wrong. She was sure she was reacting to the metal in the total knee prosthesis, but the first doctor disagreed.

She eventually went to a different orthopedic surgeon, who said she was likely having a reaction to the implant, and he recommended she have it removed to get rid of any infection. My mom followed the physician's instructions, had the metal implant removed, and a spacer was placed in her knee. This temporary cement spacer replaced the much larger knee implant. This spacer was treated with antibiotics and left in for several weeks. My mom was able to bend her knee partially and could walk with a walker for fifty to a hundred feet at a time. When the physician felt it was safe to replace the prosthesis, my mother had yet another major surgery to replace the temporary spacer with the second permanent total knee implant.

I was surprised to find out that these revisions of both total knee and total hip had been on the rise over the last decade. A common thought back in the day was that a revision would potentially be necessary if the total joint wore out over time. However, even though many knee and hip replacements turn out just fine, revision of these procedures had been starting to climb significantly over the years, and it wasn't simply due to younger people having these surgeries and the replacement wearing out, though, as you will see later, younger people are turning to replacements more so than ever before. On the contrary, the most common reason for hip and knee replacement revision is infection, especially within the first five years. Metal hypersensitivity can also be a cause of revision, though it is considered rare and often ignored, like it was in my mom's case. It occurs mostly in women and most often with total knee replacements.

Another interesting fact is that the medical community is expecting that complications resulting in revision will be rising over time. For example, one study reports that the projected incidence of knee and hip replacement revision is expected to increase by 137 percent and 601 percent from 2005 to 2030.

> ### What Percentage of People are Dissatisfied with Their Total Joint Replacement?
>
> Recent research is starting to keep track of how many patients actually regret having their total joint replacements. Typically, more people who had total knee replacements than hip replacements regret having the procedures done. And one study found that anywhere from 6 to 30 percent of patients regret having their knee replaced, and up to 14 percent of people reported dissatisfaction with their total hip replacement within five years of having it done.

What About Bone on Bone: Doesn't It Require Surgery?

Nearly once a week, a patient comes into my office, or we receive a call from a prospective patient asking if we can help with bone-on-bone pain.

The conversation typically goes something like this.

Patient: My doctor diagnosed my joint as 'bone on bone' and I need to have surgery. Can your treatment help me?

Provider: Let's first talk about the phrase 'bone on bone.' It's not a medical term or diagnosis, but it's used often when describing that on the X-ray, there isn't much space between the two bones of your joint. It isn't typically literal, meaning the bones are not actually touching each other. If they were, you wouldn't be able to put weight on that joint at all without debilitating pain.

Patient: But my doctor said it was 'bone on bone.'

Provider: Yes, we hear that all the time, but it is not accurate for the vast majority of people. What 'bone on bone' describes for most patients is a narrowing of the joint space between two bones and likely severe osteoarthritis. It's only in very rare instances that the bones would actually be rubbing together. In your hip, it's the narrowing between the femur (thigh bone) and the acetabulum (part of the pelvis that the hip connects to). In your knee, it's the narrowing of the space between the thigh bone (femur) and the leg bone (tibia). It's the same for most joints.

Patient: So, do I need surgery?

Provider: Surgery should be the last resort when nonsurgical interventions fail.

Patient: Can you help me?

Provider: Come on in for our trial and we will see if you are a good candidate for our treatment.

Is Surgery Always Necessary for Joints That Are Bone-on-Bone?

When patients hear the phrase "bone on bone," they think it means bones are rubbing up against each other, and that it's the end of the road. They think that their only option is surgery or more cortisone injections.

But most people don't understand that the description "bone on bone" is not literal, and it is not a diagnosis. If you put 'bone on bone' in any medical research database like Pub Med, zero studies come up.

Because this term is so popular, and people are told 'there isn't anything else you can do except surgery,' the average person may even have the misconception that exercise may actually make their knee worse by rubbing the bones together more. For the vast majority of cases, this is not true. Exercise, done correctly and prescribed individually to the patient's tolerance and abilities, can protect the joint and decrease joint pain. As a matter of fact, inactivity, i.e., not exercising, has been shown to negatively affect cartilage in joints. Therefore, it is imperative that even with advanced arthritis that patients are instructed in a personalized exercise program to help support pain relief and if possible, slow or eliminate the advancement of damage on the joint surfaces.

New research is showing that the narrowing of the joint space related to arthritis may be due to other factors than simply wear and tear. We will discuss each of these new breakthroughs in Part 2 of *The Pain-Free Formula*.

What About Spinal Surgery?

Studies have shown that spinal surgeries have a failure rate of anywhere between 10 and 46 percent. This includes fusions or other types of back surgery. Despite this failure rate, over 900,000 low back surgeries were performed in the early 2000s. Other research reveals that 5 to 36 percent of people who had a procedure called a discectomy to address a herniated disc in their lower back experienced leg and back pain again within two years after surgery.

What's the Cause of these Failure Rates?

Opinions abound regarding why there are failure rates of this size for those undergoing spinal surgery. Without a doubt, the spine with its many joints, close proximity to the spinal cord, and the many tentacles of nerves that arise from it and travel throughout the body, making it one of the most complex systems we have. So, finding the right structures to perform surgery on to address the chronic pain is a challenge even after extensive imaging.

Hip pain can result from the back, or back pain can result from the hip. The pelvic floor, a group of muscles in your pelvis, can contribute to back pain. Misalignment of the spine can contribute to pain, as well as disc bulges, herniations, and cysts along the spine. And to complicate matters further, the results that are seen on an MRI or X-ray could show a potential issue, like my knee showed extensive arthritis, but those issues may not be the cause of the pain someone is experiencing.

As a matter of fact, research shows that less than 5 to 10 percent of lower back pain is due to an issue with the spine.

A particularly interesting study had people without back pain undergo an MRI to look for any pathologies. Of these people, eighty percent of fifty-year-olds who showed disc degeneration had no back pain. Sixty percent of fifty-year-olds had disc bulges, and 36 percent had disc protrusion. And again, none of these individuals complained of back pain.

I myself have three levels in my lumbar spine that have bulging discs, and when I follow through with what I know I need to do, I have no pain at all.

Some people could argue that because I believe in the steps that I follow (which you will learn in Part 2), this is why it works for me. That's called the placebo effect.

What Is the Placebo Effect?

The placebo effect occurs when a patient experiences real improvement in symptoms after a sham intervention, i.e., medication, procedure, or surgery, where the sham intervention mimics the actual treatment but doesn't involve any therapeutic action. For example, in sham surgery, the patient is usually cut into, but no intervention takes place.

This placebo effect is powerful because it highlights how a patient's expectations and beliefs can influence their perception of pain and recovery. In studies comparing real surgeries to placebo surgeries, both groups often report similar levels of pain relief, suggesting that the belief in the surgery's effectiveness (not to mention the rest and rehab that follows) can trigger the body's natural healing processes. More effort should be spent finding out why people are reacting better to placebo interventions than the actual treatment.

And when you get better after doing something besides surgery, some physicians tell their patients that what they were doing probably did not make any difference, and they would have gotten better anyway.

That's hard to swallow, especially for patients experiencing chronic pain for years who finally started feeling better after applying the techniques from Part 2 of this book. But I have never heard a physician say (yet) when a patient gets better after surgery that they would likely have gotten better without the surgery. Usually, the surgery is given all the credit. But is that always true?

Placebo Surgery: Could Surgeries Be a Sham?

Imagine undergoing surgery, only to find out later that the procedure you trusted to heal your chronic pain never actually happened. This isn't science fiction—it's a reality uncovered by research into placebo, or 'sham,' surgeries. In fact, studies have shown that in more than half of these cases, patients who believed they had real surgery experienced just as much relief as those who underwent the actual procedure. The implications are profound, challenging our understanding of how much of our healing might come from the mind rather than the scalpel.

Placebos Strengthen Studies

Adding a placebo to a research project and blinding the patient and the provider as to who is receiving the placebo or the actual prevention is considered to add strength to the study's outcome, especially if the outcome is better for the group that had the surgery, pill, or procedure in comparison to the placebo group.

In a placebo surgery, only the skin or an orifice is penetrated, and no therapeutic intervention is performed.

Interestingly enough, research related to sham or placebo surgeries involving patients with pain, according to a meta-analysis of randomized, sham-controlled trials considered to have high levels of evidence, showed that in over 50 percent of the cases, the placebo group did just as well after the sham surgery than the patients who had the actual surgery.

This means that more than half of the people who thought they had the actual surgery but did not felt as good as the people who actually had the surgery!

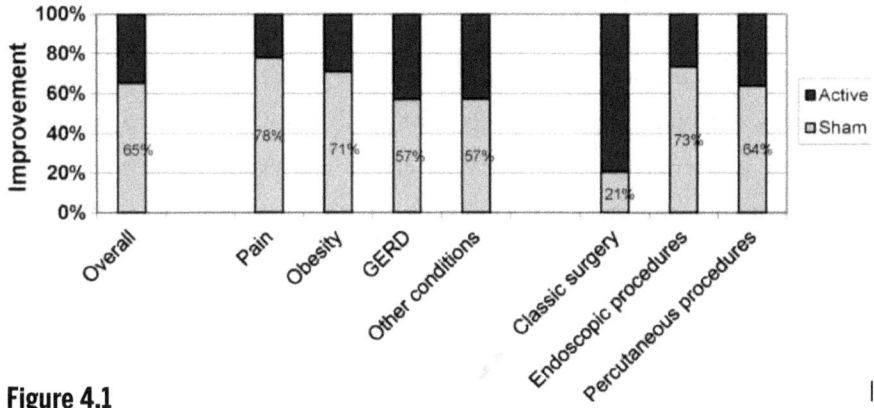

Figure 4.1

Showing improvement for those who had an active or sham surgery. Active is when the procedure was performed, and sham is when only the skin or an orifice was penetrated, and no therapeutic intervention was performed.

This type of placebo response was noted in over fifty-five studies with over 3,500 patients that were "randomized controlled trials of surgery and invasive procedures that penetrated the skin or an orifice and had a parallel sham procedure for comparison."

But even more stunning, when you look at Figure 4.1 you can see when surgeries that were not specifically related to pain are removed, a **whopping 78 percent of patients undergoing the placebo or sham surgery for pain (fifteen studies with over 1,500 people) had improvement. This means the majority of those who experienced improvement in their symptoms were in the placebo/sham group! In other words, only those who had a general anesthetic and who were cut open for surgery but received *no* true surgical intervention experienced the most improvement when compared to the number of people who received the actual therapeutic intervention.** Most of these surgeries were related to low back pain knee arthritis, or meniscus repairs. All of these patients would likely have had positive findings on their MRI or X-rays of some physical issue that was seemingly causing them pain. But even more than 75 percent of the patients who did *not* have the issue addressed with surgery got better.

This research is why, in recent years, there have been less arthroscopic surgeries for knee meniscus repairs and diffuse low back pain. I am guessing, in turn, that this is why we are seeing a significant increase in total joint replacements in younger populations.

Joint Replacements Shift to a Younger Demographic

Patients who in the past would have had an arthroscopic (scope) surgery to 'clean out' the knee or to repair a meniscus are now being sent to physical therapy, or simply told by their physician that he or she won't do the surgery because research shows that the surgeries are not better than placebo.

That must have been a big loss of revenue for hospitals. It would make sense then that joint replacements were considered earlier to keep operating rooms active. I rarely if ever saw a knee or hip replacement in someone younger than sixty-five when I first started practicing. The reason was always that the replacement had a certain lifetime, so physicians wanted patients to wait as long as possible to have their joints replaced.

But more recently, according to the American Academy of Orthopedic Surgeons, knee replacements and hip replacements increased 188 percent and 123 percent respectively in patients aged forty-five to sixty-four from 2000 to 2009. This was the same period that the sham surgeries were shown to be better than the real intervention. In that same period, for those sixty-five to eighty-four, the total knee and hip replacements increased 89 percent and 54 percent respectively.

It has been happening with shoulders, as well. Sham surgeries regarding labral repairs, biceps tenodesis, acromial decompression, and bone spur removal performed just as good or better than the actual surgical intervention. And curiously, American Academy of Orthopedic Surgeons (AAOS) reported that about 18,000 total shoulder replacements (TSR) were performed in the US in the year 2000. By 2017, 823,361 TSR were performed in the United States. And by 2040, there is expected to be a 700 percent increase of TSR performed in the US.

Coincidence? I will let you be the judge.

To be fair, procedures and the implants have likely improved during this time. One could argue that yes, they have, but at the same time the number of revisions and complications have risen as well.

Sham Surgeries vs. Total Joint Replacements

Interestingly enough, no sham versus active study appears to exist to evaluate whether the high cost and significant pain, and loss of income from time off a patient experiences after a total joint replacement surgery would be any better than a placebo surgery.

A research journal article makes an interesting comment: "... roughly four out of five patients declare they are satisfied postoperatively, justifying the procedure's frequency and high costs. It is sobering to realize, however, that the evidence base in favor of this procedure remains circumstantial."

You only have to watch a few *Law and Order* episodes to understand what "circumstantial" means.

In this context, circumstantial evidence refers to indirect signs that suggest a procedure might be effective, like patients reporting satisfaction after surgery. However, this satisfaction doesn't directly prove the surgery works; it could be due to the placebo effect or other factors. The statement highlights that while many patients are happy with the results, there is no solid, direct proof that the procedure itself is the reason for their improvement.

The study's authors go on to say, "We believe that after five decades, we must hold surgical procedures to the same standard we apply to medications—these interventions (joint replacements) must be subjected to a placebo-controlled randomized trial. Millions of patients deserve the answer to this question."

It will definitely be interesting to see if that ever happens.

Surgery or No Surgery?

Considering the significant evidence that some surgeries for chronic pain aren't better than placebo, how do you know what to do? Should you have surgery or not?

As you can see, the evidence often shows that surgeries for chronic conditions may not be a great option, and most physicians would agree that they should not be the first option. But since you have read through these first four chapters which delineate that surgeries, typical injections such as cortisone, and oral medications are often not the answer, the fact remains: you are in pain.

How, then, are you supposed to address that pain?

How can you make it go away without medication, injections, or surgery?

Part 2 of *The Pain-Free Formula* will provide you with a systemic approach to assessing and addressing the true root cause of your pain.

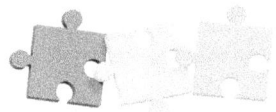

Key Pieces

Surgery as a Last Resort: Unless it is an emergency, surgery, especially for chronic pain, should not be the first option. Evidence suggests that many surgeries might not offer better outcomes than placebo procedures.

Rise in Unnecessary Surgeries: There is a growing concern about the increasing rates of unnecessary surgeries, particularly in younger demographics, driven by outdated or circumstantial evidence.

Understanding 'Bone on Bone': The term 'bone on bone' is often misleading. It doesn't always necessitate surgery, and alternative treatments should be considered first, as they can be very effective.

Joint Replacement Concerns: Joint replacements are becoming more common, even in younger patients, despite increasing rates of dissatisfaction and the potential for complications or revisions. And there are no placebo-controlled studies related to joint replacements to see if, in fact, they have better results than a placebo.

NOTE: I am not against surgery, and at times, I refer patients to physicians to have an overall assessment and determine to the best of their ability whether surgery is the best choice. But I am against patients not receiving all the information they need to make the best decision for themselves, including not giving patients information about alternative treatment options. There are many less invasive or noninvasive options that are successful.

PART TWO
The New Pain Paradigm
A BLUEPRINT TO LASTING PAIN RELIEF

> "Do the best you can until you know better. Then when you know better, do better."
>
> –Maya Angelou

It was a Saturday afternoon and, if I am being honest, I was not excited to be seeing patients that day. I had a full load of classes in my nursing program, and I was absolutely exhausted. I also had an exam on Monday that I needed to study for.

But Anne was my last patient, so there was a light at the end of the tunnel. I hoped that she hadn't sensed my restlessness. She was seeing me for a pelvic health condition called dyspareunia (pronounced dis-pa-runia). In other words, she was experiencing pain with sexual intercourse. We went through the evaluation where I asked her more in-depth questions based on the answers she had filled in on her intake form. This was followed by an internal assessment where I palpate (a medical term that means 'examine by touch') the muscles of the pelvic floor to see if I can create the pain that she normally feels.

I also checked the strength and flexibility of her hips, low back, legs, and even her feet. We talked about chronic pain (she had been experiencing pain with intercourse for over five years), and I instructed her in diaphragmatic breathing exercises. These types of breathing exercises are supported by research at renowned institutes such as John's Hopkins Hospital as an adjunct to pain relief, and then I explained our SoftWave technology to her that you will learn about in Chapter 7. And after giving her final consent, we then treated her pelvic floor with SoftWave, followed that with manual therapy, i.e., treating trigger points discovered in the assessment. She was stunned at how much better her symptoms were when we did the final assessment of her trigger points at the end of the treatment.

As I sat on the side of the padded table where she was lying flat, covered in our sheets to maintain her privacy and keep her warm, we made eye contact. Before I left the room to let my office manager know what the plan was for the next treatment, I noticed that Anne's eyes had welled up with tears.

"Anne," I asked softly and gently placed my hand on her arm, "are you okay?"

She nodded slowly and silently as a tear trickled down the side of her temple.

"I think maybe this is a good time to practice the breathing that we talked about."

She smiled meekly and took a deep breath. Her right hand over her abdomen rose and fell back to its original position.

"That's great, Anne. You got it," I said.

She repeated the breath three more times.

After the third breath, she wiggled up onto her elbows. I took the hint and raised the head of the padded table so that she was able to sit up.

I looked up into her blinking blue eyes. She gently rubbed the outside of her eye with the edge of her index finger, and I noticed some red blotching on her neck.

"How are you feeling?" I asked.

Not sure if she was ready to reply, I sat silently. Then she spoke.

"I'm fine. I just..." she paused and looked straight ahead of her. "I am just so grateful," she said, and she took another deep breath.

I kept quiet.

"I'm just so grateful that you took all that time with me. It really seems like you care, and you actually want me to get better."

Now it was my turn. I felt a lump in my throat as I teared up.

"Oh, gosh, you are so welcome," I said, blinking incessantly.

Our eyes met again, and I blurted out, "I'm not crying, you're crying!" And we both laughed.

"Seriously though," she was sounding like herself again, "that was so thorough." She swung her legs over the side of the table and her feet dangled in mid-air. "I have been to so many doctors and places to have treatments. The last place I went for therapy, they basically gave me a sheet with some exercises on it and talked me through the diagrams. Then they told me to go home and do the exercises three times a day. I still have no idea if I am doing them right."

The wheels on my rolling stool rumbled, as I cruised toward the desk and grabbed a tissue box. Better late than never.

I reached out toward Anne, and she pulled one out of the box, wiped her nose, and continued. "I went to see them three times, and it was pretty much the same thing every time. And my doctor only had about ten minutes to spend with me." After blowing her nose and taking one more big breath in and exhaling it out, she concluded, "so yeah, thank you."

"Thank you for your kind words. That truly means a lot. I am sorry you had that experience, but I am glad you found us."

I stood up and asked if she was okay again. She nodded definitively and I walked toward the door. As I pulled it closed behind me, I was not sure what I felt.

It's times like these when I experience a mix of emotions. I was definitely touched that Anne verbalized her appreciation and recognized that I tried to be as thorough as possible in my evaluation to assess the cause of her pain. But under the surface, a familiar irritation burned in my chest. Anne experienced what many are experiencing today in my profession. I was growing more and more frustrated hearing about this cookie-cutter care that includes basically an exercise sheet, and not much else. There are many reasons for this, in my opinion, substandard care, but the one most glaring cause is declining reimbursement from insurance companies, resulting in clinics having to see multiple people in an hour just to make the same or even less revenue than they made the year before. Back in the day, care was typically one-on-one; today in larger insurance-based clinics, one-on-one care is a rare find and often limited to those dealing with more sensitive issues such as pelvic pain.

Anne left and I locked up. As I drove home, not looking forward to studying for my exam, I began to appreciate why our clinic has gotten busier and busier over the years, despite being fee-for-service and patients needing to pay out-of-pocket for their treatment.

Part of it is quality and quantity of care. Patients appreciate spending adequate time with their provider. We spend thirty minutes to an hour, at times, on one-on-one care. Time is often what the typical physician and now PT doesn't have.

But the other part, which is more of a concern for me as I look at how the medical profession has changed over the years, is the lack of digging deep enough to find the underlying cause or trigger of symptoms like pain. You've seen in the previous chapters how medications and potentially unnecessary procedures are by far becoming the norm in our medical system today. And why is that? There is little effort placed on truly interviewing and listening to a patient, often due to large time and budget constraints, and there's even less time spent looking for the true underlying cause of the patient's symptoms. Conventional medicine spends more time covering up the symptoms with a quick fix like medications or familiar injections, potentially resulting in long-term issues, rather than searching for the true cause.

Don't get me wrong though, if I am bleeding out in a car accident, I don't want to go to a local shaman. Take me to the emergency room and let them put me back together. Emergency medicine is amazing and has saved countless lives in the last century. And there's no doubt that medications such as antibiotics have done the same, but even those have been overused to the point that our bodies are becoming resistant to certain medications, so when we need them the most, they may not work.

But related to chronic muscle and joint pain, along with other medical diagnoses, problems occur when short- or long-term treatment is just masking the symptoms and isn't addressing the underlying trigger (whether tangible or intangible) or the root cause of the pain. This masking often results in more medications and more procedures to treat the side effects of the first or second treatment.

Case in point: cortisone injections, as discussed, are an invasive treatment that has been used for years to address joint pain. They have now been related to more degeneration in joints and tears in muscles/tendons, but because they are covered by insurance, several million of these injections are given per year in the United States, despite the research showing the potential harm they cause.

Based on my experience, I've seen too many patients receive inadequate treatment and attention from professionals. While there are excellent providers, and I refer patients outside my scope to the best providers I can find, major changes are needed in the healthcare system. Though out of the scope of this book to discuss, it is crystal clear to patients that to providers need more time for assessment and treatment of their patients as well as education about options other than surgery, drugs or injections.

In the second half of this book, I hope the information provided helps you change this paradigm, so Anne's experience is more the norm than the exception. If you are a practitioner under the grind of seeing three to four or more patients in an hour, see what you can do to change that. If you are a patient stuck in a system that is only able to churn patients out without digging deep for the reason you are having your symptoms, look outside your insurance coverage for care. In addition, there are many extremely talented providers out there who just don't have all the answers for patients whose pain has not resolved via conventional means. My hope is that the following information also helps them.

Start with finding the underlying causes or triggers of your pain. Part Two of *The Pain-Free Formula* is dedicated to educating patients like you and providers looking for unconventional answers about the underlying cause(s) or trigger(s) of chronic pain. Armed with this information, you can seek out the care that is best for you when:

- Conventional medicine isn't working for you
- You've tried everything and nothing has worked
- You want alternative solutions backed by research which don't involve more medications, surgeries, and injections

Welcome to Part Two of The Pain-Free Formula.

Note: The chapters that follow are not meant to be looked at as an either/or scenario. There is a greater likelihood that your issue with pain, especially if it's chronic, is related to not just one but some or several topics in the following chapters. And remember, these suggestions are not meant to diagnose, cure, or treat any disease. The information is educational only. Please always discuss any changes or treatments with your healthcare provider.

CHAPTER 5

Why Won't My Pain Go Away?

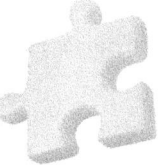

"Perseverance is failing nineteen times and succeeding the twentieth."

–Julie Andrews

Sarah had always been active, enjoying long hikes and weekend tennis matches. However, over the past year, after her last regional doubles match, she had begun to experience a dull, persistent ache in her knee. Initially, she brushed it off, assuming it was just a minor injury that would heal on its own. But the pain lingered, gradually becoming a constant companion that affected her daily activities.

Frustrated and seeking answers, Sarah visited her doctor. The initial examination and X-rays showed no significant issues, so an MRI was ordered. The results came back that her medial meniscus was torn, and an arthroscopic knee surgery would be the likely step if a course of physical therapy wasn't successful in addressing her knee pain. The meniscus tear, based on where Sarah felt her pain, and the special tests performed confirmed the meniscus was likely the trigger of her current complaints.

What do I mean by trigger?

A trigger is any stimulus, event, or factor that activates or intensifies inflammation or the experience of pain.

.Tangible Triggers: Obvious Offenders

- An action, movement, or structure
- Continues to irritate connective tissue (bone, tendons, ligaments, meniscus, fascia) or muscle
- It is tangible, i.e., it can be measured, palpated, or observed. Damage to these tissues can often be seen on tests such as MRI, CAT scan, or X-ray.

The most obvious example of a tangible trigger related to pain would be a broken bone or fracture. This can usually be seen on an X-ray. Its presence is clearly the cause of pain at the site of the fracture.

Other examples of tangible triggers that cause pain are structures that are damaged from an injury, overuse, or both. In Sarah's case, it was the medial meniscus. But it could be partially torn ligaments, inflamed tendons, a muscle strain, or other torn or irritated structures such as a labral tear in the shoulder or hip. These tangible triggers of pain typically occur consistently only with certain movements and can be identified by the providers performing special tests that involve moving the body part a certain way to determine if that movement or 'special test' elicits the same pain the patient experiences.

Movements that continue to irritate these inflamed structures, or the fact that structures such as the labrum or meniscus have poor blood supply and are prone to having difficulty healing, can often keep tissues from completing the body's innate healing process.

Without continued triggering of the damaged tissue, the inflammatory process should allow healing to take place and pain to resolve. Our body performs this miraculous recovery process every single day constantly, whether it is bruised tissue that we can see changing back to normal tissue over time or internally, when the body heals structures that we are not consciously aware of, such as abrasions on our blood vessels, irritation to our gut from foods we eat, or replacing cells that are damaged or old from wear and tear with healthy replicas. The inflammatory process is an internal factory that is constantly humming along, keeping us around to see another day. See the illustration below.

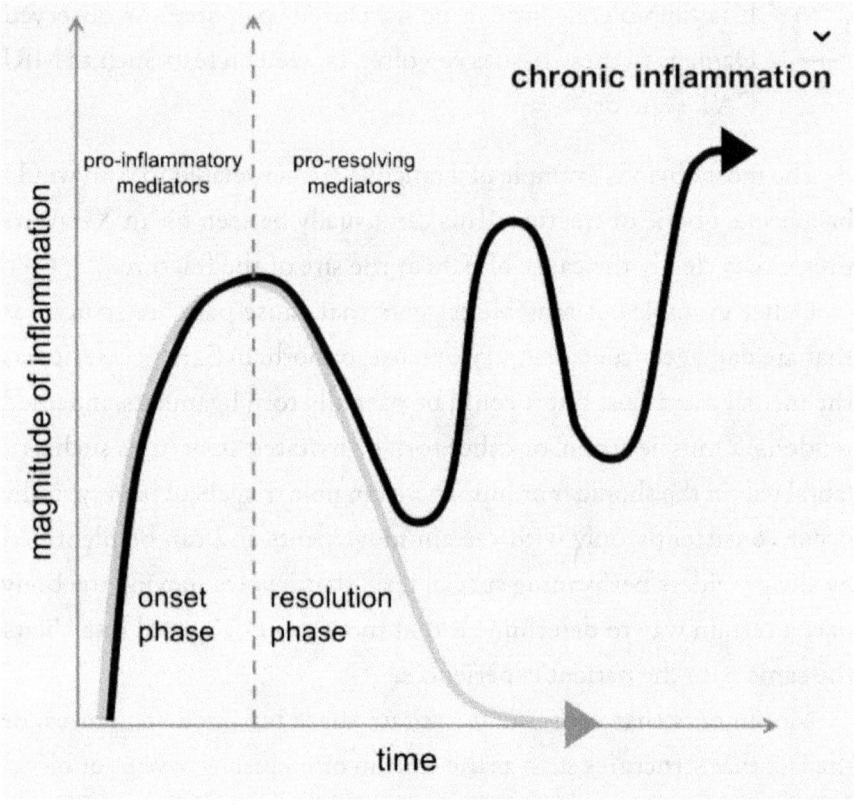

Figure 5.1 The Inflammatory Process

This image shows the onset and resolution of the inflammation process initiated and completed by our immune system. Inflammation occurs after an injury, irritation to an area, or simply as a part of normal cellular turnover. It starts when pro-inflammatory mediators such as M1 macrophages release cytokines (e.g., IL-1) and travel to the area to begin the healing process. These molecules begin or restart inflammation.

The resolution phase consists of the pro-resolving mediators working, also known as anti-inflammatory mediators. Examples of these would be M2 macrophages. These molecules can release a substance to enable stem cells, another anti-inflammatory mediatory, to grow. These and other pro-resolving mediators must be present for the body's innate healing process to resolve the crisis and heal the tissue. Or, at the very least, decrease the inflammation to the point that it is not felt as pain and hopefully does not interfere with function.

More simply put, the pro-inflammatory molecules that come from the activation of our immune system are the first responders on the scene. Whether there is an irritation to the skin, a torn ligament, or an inflamed tendon, this is how the healing process begins. After the immune system starts the pro-inflammatory phase, the body segues into the anti-inflammatory phase, and if triggers are removed, the irritation stops, and the tissue can fully heal.

For example, in Chapter 3, in the section subtitled "Inflammation 101," I talked about having a scratch on my hand. It starts out looking red and puffy. If I don't leave it alone, and I continue to scratch it ten times a day. This trigger (me scratching the injured area) will perpetuate the pro-inflammatory process and keep the area irritated, often painful, and slow to heal. The same goes for pain in a joint or other connective tissue. For example, someone with plantar fasciitis who wears poor footwear has tight calf muscles or both, often creates forces that cause the arch of the foot to fall inward. This movement i.e. the biomechanics of their foot while walking (tangible trigger #1) continuously stretches that fascia while continuously irritating the tissue and triggering a repetitive pro-inflammatory response.

If you have pain with activity or after resting for a while and then when trying to resume activity the pain continues, this could be a sign of a tangible trigger perpetuating the pro-inflammatory process. For example, it's quite common for those with plantar fasciitis to have pain in the first few minutes of a walk, but then as the tissues warm up a bit, the pain dissipates or goes away. But that first step after a long sleep or getting up after sitting for a while feels like a hot poker or sharp knife digging into the bottom of their heel. This pain in the morning results from the fascia at the bottom of the foot being shortened all night as the foot relaxes during sleep. Then when the person wakes up and puts weight on the foot, they stretch that shortened irritated tissue abruptly and pain ensues. Plantar fasciitis as a whole can be a result of poor shoe wear or faulty biomechanics of the hip, knee, foot, or ankle. Decreased flexibility, decreased strength, and hormone changes can contribute to this, as well. These are all tangible triggers that can be observed or measured and subsequently corrected to help eliminate the pain.

The same goes for any joint that continues to hurt after a reasonable recovery period. If the biomechanics (how muscles, bones, tendons, and ligaments work together to move the body) are putting stress on an area, especially after an old or new injury, inflammation and, subsequently, pain can be triggered by irritation of the tissue. If the trigger is not addressed or removed altogether or lessened, then the irritation/inflammation and resulting pain will likely continue. Interventions such as physical therapy by skilled practitioners can remove these tangible triggers by addressing biomechanics. This relieves the stress on the joint or muscle and can result in the elimination of pain if the patient's immune system, described above, is healthy and supports the healing process.

Intangible Triggers: The Subtle Saboteurs

Now that you know about tangible triggers, it's time to learn about triggers of pain that aren't always as easily observed or measured. These intangible triggers are often the culprits causing persistent pain, especially if pain continues after the tangible triggers have been addressed. Finding and eliminating the intangible trigger, is often the key to being pain-free.

What are intangible triggers?

- Hidden patterns or processes in the body, such as neurological signals, that can keep pain recurring, even when there's no clear evidence of new or ongoing damage at the original injury site or the area where you feel pain
- Often not observed on an MRI, CAT scan, or X-ray, or if noted, doesn't appear to be significant.
- Can't be observed during movement or during assessment of joint biomechanics.

Some blood tests may be able to give an indication that an intangible trigger, such as systemic inflammation, is present, but it's not always specific as to where that inflammation is based. For example, blood tests such as C-Reactive Protein (CRP), Erythrocyte Sedimentation Rate (ESR), or lactate dehydrogenase (LDH) when elevated can indicate general inflammation or muscle damage respectively, but it doesn't typically narrow down where that damage can be found.

- Antibodies related to autoimmune issues are another sign that intangible triggers of inflammation are present in the body.

Intangible and tangible triggers can be present at the same time. This is where the solution and treatment must be multifaceted to fully address and eliminate pain. Unfortunately, with regard to muscle and joint pain, our conventional approach tends to be geared only toward fixing potential tangible triggers with surgery or addressing any known or unknown trigger with drugs or injections, which are often designed to suppress symptoms and not address the root cause of the issue.

Addressing the underlying cause is akin to finding the right puzzle piece or pieces to eliminate the pain, instead of covering it up. This is the challenge for both practitioner and patient.

Systemic vs. Localized Inflammation

At times, an injury may occur, and the pain may continue due to a tangible trigger, i.e., weak hip muscles can cause the knee to turn in. When the knee turns, the arch of the foot can turn in, and these movements, if excessive, could result in hip pain, knee pain, and/or foot pain. This pain and inflammation would be localized to a certain area.

But what happens if this localized inflammation, which may be triggered initially by an injury to an area, is present while the body is also overwhelmed with systemic inflammation, i.e., the body is generally inflamed from conditions such as obesity, diabetes, autoimmune issues, fibromyalgia, or even gut issues?

Researchers hypothesize, based on credible, evidence-based research, that systemic inflammation (often present due to intangible trigger(s)) can exacerbate localized inflammation, cause fibrosis, and make it very difficult for the body to complete the healing process. See Figure 5.2.

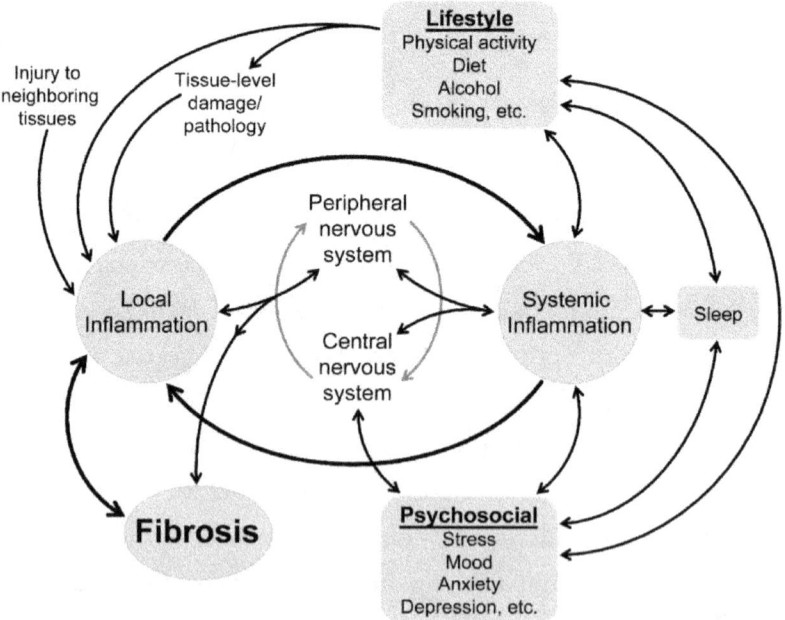

Figure 5.2 Fibrosis can result from localized and/or systemic inflammation.

Fibrosis in Figure 5.2 relates to thickening, hardening, or scarring of tissues due to a build-up of collagen. Injuries to tendons, ligaments, menisci, and other structures can lead to fibrosis, resulting in chronic pain. Later, we will discuss the occurrence of both systemic and localized inflammation in more detail and how to address it, but the purpose of mentioning this here is to illustrate that the presence of systemic inflammation associated with autoimmune diseases, gut issues, obesity, diabetes, or other chronic, systemic diseases can result in the exacerbation of localized inflammation (here illustrated as fibrosis) after a joint or muscle injury, exhibiting how both intangible and tangible triggers can create and perpetuate muscle and joint pain.

NOTE: This systemic inflammation doesn't always result from the disease processes listed above. A transition in our hormones can contribute to this as well.

A Hormonal Connection to Joint and Muscle Pain

I often learn more about alternative causes of joint and muscle pain from patients who have come to me for other reasons.

Catherine was no exception. She was entering menopause, but not quite there yet. She had skipped four or five months of periods, and gradually started experiencing a common symptom many women have: hot flashes. She experienced them more at night than during the day. Some evenings, Catherine would wake up drenched in sweat and end up throwing the covers off and having to change her pajama top because she was soaked to the skin. She and her husband would argue about what temperature the thermometer should be set at. One would have a fan and the other would have three blankets. Catherine was dealing with this issue night after night when she saw me to help her address her menopausal issues with functional medicine.

What I haven't told you so far about Catherine is that she is a personal friend of mine. So, at times, it was a strain on our friendship if she asked for my advice but ended up ignoring it. Because she would hear me over and over, albeit gently, I thought about what she needed to do for her situation.

She typically blamed it on her stress and lack of sleep . . . after all, Catherine had five children ranging from ages ten to twenty-two. Stress was definitely a factor in her life. And as many of us do, Catherine just put that behind her as something she did not have control over because of all the craziness in her schedule day to day. She was convinced she would just have to live with it and continue to fantasize about running away to a beach and burying herself in a favorite book without phones, emails, or constant requests from the people she loved.

In our consultation, we discussed her hormone levels changing as she approached the cessation of her periods, and how that was one type of stress on her system that could account for her hot flashes. This is often exacerbated by emotional, physiological, or physical stress.

Our goal was to assess and address the shift in hormones naturally and then see what other symptoms were left. The personalized program that we put together decreased the hot flashes significantly, but the muscle aches and pains in her neck and shoulders persisted. I suggested that she go to her primary care physician to check the level of specific hormones in her system. Her physician, unfortunately, did only one of the five blood tests that I had recommended. The tests came back within the range, and the physician told her she was "perfectly normal," a common response. And though he could unequivocally tell her what the problem wasn't, he did not have any explanation as to what the problem was and what she could do about it.

When my patients get to this point in their consultations with their physicians, I will often suggest other avenues to get testing done. Direct primary care clinics and franchises like Any Lab Test Now are often good alternatives. Online options such as canaryclub.org also exist. Patients can usually request the blood tests they want from these companies, or we order urinary tests to determine issues not often looked at by conventionally trained doctors.

Thankfully, there are several steps you will learn about later in Part 2 that patients can take to address muscle and joint pain while avoiding the development of a full-blown autoimmune disease, improving thyroid function, and optimizing sex hormones such as estrogen, progesterone, and testosterone. But is there anything else besides these sex hormones and aforementioned disease processes that could be considered triggers?

The Gut-Joint Axis

Other examples of intangible triggers contributing to systemic inflammation causing chronic pain are foods we eat that negatively impact our gut. A clear example of this is patients with celiac disease (CD). CD is an autoimmune disease. A person with CD is intolerant to gluten-containing foods. It's much more prevalent today than in the past few decades.

My patient Susan had come to see me for functional medicine support because she was having difficulty getting pregnant. However, in our evaluation, Susan listed her issues with joint pain. She did not mention anything about digestive issues, and interestingly enough, 21 percent of those with CD don't have any digestive complaints. This is referred to as subclinical celiac disease.

Susan reported "normal" flatulence and regularly formed bowel movements. When I questioned her about the joint pain she reported, her response was that it wasn't a result of any injury she could remember. But randomly, she would be sit and watch television, and her joints would ache. This could happen any time throughout the day, and often at night. She felt tired frequently and lacked energy, as well. Pardon the pun, but my gut was telling me to send her to be tested for celiac disease.

The blood tests showed there was a strong possibility that she had it. She went on to have an endoscopy. This involved having a tube inserted down her throat to see if there was, in fact, damage to structures of her small intestine called villi, a common finding in those with celiac disease. The doctor said the damage to her gut was severe. He rated it as an eight on a scale of zero to ten. The diagnosis of celiac disease was confirmed. When I saw Susan three months later, she had given up gluten completely. Gluten-containing foods must be eliminated if a person has celiac disease. And after stopping foods containing gluten, her joint pain went away.

Although the damage related to celiac disease begins in the small intestine, other areas of the body, such as the joints and muscles, are often affected as well. This is an example of how a trigger of inflammation from the gut can impact structures such as joints, which are away from the original site of inflammation. Research shows that those with celiac disease are more susceptible to inflammation in the structures in and around the joints and have an increased risk of osteoporosis. Osteoarthritis is also more common in adults with celiac disease. More and more gut issues are being connected to joint and muscle pain.

But food intolerances such as celiac disease aren't the only gut issues that can cause joint pain. Food sensitivities play a major role. We will talk about more of these triggers in detail in the coming chapters.

The Brain, Pain, and Intangible Triggers

The next type of intangible trigger can seem a bit far-fetched when you first hear about it. Many people, including myself, find it more vague and often difficult to understand. When I first encountered it twenty years ago, it was a bit challenging to wrap my head around because it did not fit the model of what I thought I already knew about joint and muscle pain.

But experience and thirty years of watching patients continue to suffer from chronic pain when the medical establishment said they were fine has opened my eyes and mind to other possible causes of chronic pain. Thankfully, research is starting to catch up to this concept.

Now, before you close the book and say I am full of it, remember that reputable research institutions have supported the presence of this intangible trigger that originates from our mind/body connection.

Research has proven that triggers such as thoughts, beliefs, self-talk, how we process what others say to us, memories, and past experiences can contribute to pain. Jimmy is a good example. He was a twenty-one-year-old college student who was accompanied by his mother on his first visit with me. She made an appointment to address Jimmy's back pain that he had been experiencing for nearly two years. In our evaluation, we talked about everything that he had done to address the pain. He had physical therapy, kept up with his exercises, tried chiropractors, acupuncture, and pain medications, but nothing seemed to help.

His mother was concerned that the supplements he was taking as a pre- and post-workout regime were causing the pain to persist. But Jimmy explained that he had stopped those supplements at least three months prior and was still experiencing the pain, plus the pain had started well before he started taking the supplements.

With my physical evaluation, I couldn't reproduce his pain. His muscles felt completely normal to palpation, and no movements or manual therapy caused him any increased pain. Yet he continued to rate his pain as a five to eight out of ten on a zero to ten pain scale, and his relationship with his mom was visibly strained in our meeting.

On his second visit, he came on his own. As we talked through my findings from visit number one and dove a bit more into the history related to pain, I asked more about his mental health. Was he under significant stress at school or at home? He said his studies were hard but not overly stressful. When I asked about family life, he began to visibly shift in his seat. I brought up a book by Lorimer Moseley called *Pain and Perception: A Closer Look at Why We Hurt*.

Moseley, a neurobiologist and university professor, explains that pain is not just a physical sensation, but a complex and highly individual experience influenced by a variety of factors, including emotional, cognitive, and social elements. The research was related to the intangible triggers discussed here, i.e., thoughts, feelings, stress, etc.

I asked Jimmy what happened with his pain if he sat there and thought about a time at home when he felt significant stress. He shifted in his seat some more.

"What's happening to your pain right now?" I asked.

His narrowed eyes met mine as he instinctively grabbed his upper trapezius, the muscle along his upper back between his neck and shoulder and started rubbing it as he sat silently.

"Is there a change in the pain?"

His eyes softened and he slowly nodded his head.

I asked if he noticed that when he was away from those stresses, such as traveling with his friends, the pain changed.

He slowly nodded his head again.

I asked him how it changed.

"It's less," he said. "And when I am hanging with friends, sometimes it's completely gone."

As I watched the figurative lightbulb turn on in his head, his eyes widened, and he sat up straight while slowly removing his hand from his upper trap.

I asked him if he would like a referral to a local psychologist that I knew at that time who worked with adolescents and college students. He nodded one more time. I grabbed the business card from my top desk drawer and slid the card across the table, letting him know I was here if he needed any more support. A few years later, I received a message from him letting me know that he had graduated from college and was working in a bank for his first job, working out, and feeling well. He was still seeing the psychologist occasionally.

Moseley has run several experiments showing how the brain influences our experience of pain in his TEDx talk titled *Why Things Hurt*, which at the time of writing can be found on YouTube. In the talk, he discusses how these different triggers can produce pain and are related to chronic pain. "If we keep stimulating neurons that produce pain," whether it be an actual or imagined stimulus, those neurons (nerves that communicate with and within the brain) "get better at producing pain. They become more and more sensitive, and we need a smaller and smaller influence" to create the pain.

If you recall from our previous discussion about medications such as opioids and even NSAIDs and others, taking them long-term can make our physiology hypersensitive or more susceptible to feeling pain.

Intangible triggers, whether they are a result of systemic inflammation or stressors on our system, can be difficult to pin down without conscious effort, a bit of digging, and sometimes introspection. And though research supports their existence in chronic pain patients, medical professionals don't often discuss these possible triggers with patients. Or if they do, their answer to the trigger is often pain medications, anti-depressants, or anti-anxiety medications.

While all pain may be experienced or interpreted in the brain, as Moseley purports, not all pain is strictly due to emotional stress, though it is fair to note that all types of pain can be increased by it.

Thankfully, addressing chronic pain through cognitive restructuring techniques tapping into a special process in the brain called neuroplasticity can effectively address chronic pain. In Chapter 13 more will be discussed about these and other techniques.

Chronic Pain: A Blessing in Disguise?

After helping hundreds of individuals identify triggers to aid with pain relief, and experiencing significant joint and muscle pain myself, I have to admit that calling chronic pain "a blessing" may be a stretch. When you are the one dealing with disturbed sleep, minimal activity, and not being able to enjoy simple things like watching a movie on your couch or spending quality time with family and friends, it can be distressing. But the goal of these preliminary chapters has been to help you see that pain can serve a valuable purpose to protect you.

Pain, whether acute or chronic, acts as a warning system, alerting you to areas that need to be addressed, hopefully to prevent further damage, thus prompting you to take action. It's vital to heed your body's warning signals and finally address the root cause, which may lie in one or all of the systems discussed above.

Contrary to the conventional approach of masking pain with medication, surgery, or injections, addressing the root cause is the prime objective of *The Pain-Free Formula*. Rather than simply covering up the pain with the proverbial rug, seeking out solutions that promote healing at many levels and eliminating pain at its source is your gateway to relief and getting back to what you love to do.

Gone are the days of solely treating symptoms. Together, let's go forward and build the boat that can carry you to a pain-free life again.

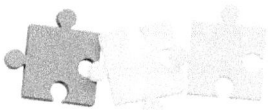

Key Pieces

Pain is a puzzle—Identifying your triggers is like finding the corner pieces, and from there you can make connections and move inward toward relief.

Identify Pain Triggers: Recognizing both tangible and intangible triggers is essential for effectively managing and resolving pain. By identifying and addressing these triggers, you can significantly accelerate your journey to pain relief.

Tangible Triggers: These are physical, measurable factors like joint injuries or inflammation, which can be seen on medical imaging or identified through physical exams.

Intangible Triggers: Harder to detect, these include factors like hormonal changes, gut health issues, or psychological stressors that can perpetuate pain even without visible damage.

Systemic vs. Localized Inflammation: Systemic inflammation from conditions like autoimmune diseases, diabetes, or a less-than-optimal eating plan can exacerbate localized injuries, making pain harder to resolve.

Pain as a Warning System: Chronic pain can be seen as the body's way of signaling deeper issues that need to be addressed at their root rather than just masking symptoms.

CHAPTER 6

Biomechanics and Insufficient Movement Patterns
A Common Tangible Trigger

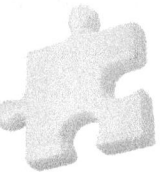

"Movement is medicine."

–Lorimer Moseley

The light shone in my bedroom window and rested its warm rays across my face, snuggled into the pillow. As my body started to become conscious along with my mind, I pushed myself up and sat at the edge of my bed. I could feel the coolness of the hardwood floors beneath my feet. With my eyes half-open, I transferred my weight forward, and as I stood up, a piercing pain at the bottom of my heel jabbed me like someone took a hot poker and shoved it in.

What the heck? I knew I had to move to the bathroom quickly, as nature was calling, but with each step, excruciating pain shot through the bottom of my foot.

I limped to the bathroom and found some relief as I sat on the cool seat, now fully awake and confused about what had just happened.

About eight months prior to this, as I detailed before, I had hurt my knee at a wedding dancing with my son. I had just been feeling better and recovered from that injury. So, what in the world was going on now?

As I sat in the bathroom, I went over and over in my head how I could have developed the pain in my heel, also known as plantar fasciitis. I had treated hundreds of patients with this issue but had not experienced it myself.

As I scrolled through the few months prior in my brain, I had to admit, I had noticed that I was walking differently since my knee incident at the wedding. My calf was tighter, and my gait pattern had changed due to the altered biomechanics in my knee following the ligament sprain. This change in how I had been walking for the previous eight months appeared to have put different stressors on my hip and foot.

Feeling a bit dejected about starting to experience yet another bout of pain, it suddenly dawned on me: one year prior, I had done a survey of one hundred women who had experienced plantar fasciitis. I did this while I creating my online program, the Foot Pain Relief System, to help those dealing with persistent plantar fasciitis recover. (Email info@newyouhealthandwellness.com for more information.)

To find out what women with this issue wanted to know, I created a ten-question survey asking them about their experience with plantar fasciitis, as well as their circumstances and health leading up to the onset of their foot and heel pain.

Sixty percent of women surveyed recalled a previous injury to their lower extremity within one to two years of developing plantar fasciitis. Now, sitting on my porcelain throne, that made complete sense to me. When you have an injury in your knee, hip, or even your back, you will undoubtedly end up compensating due to the pain. This change in my gait persisted even after the injury healed.

Walking or moving differently due to an injury to a joint can put a new type of pressure on other areas of the body, forcing muscles and joints to work differently than perhaps they ever have. This change can also stress tissues beneath the surface, such as fascia, the tissue beneath the skin that wraps around every muscle and organ in the body. If this is disrupted or stressed in a way it hasn't been before, other issues can pop up as a result, especially during a hormonal transition such as pregnancy, perimenopause, or post-menopause.

This would be a perfect example of a localized tangible trigger. My heel pain was most probably triggered by the change in the way I was walking secondary to my previous knee injury. This is called compensation. As a result of this compensation, the biomechanics of my leg changed, resulting in stress being put on tissues that had not been stressed that way before. Over time, this can result in pain that happens gradually as a result of tangible triggers.

What are Biomechanics?

Biomechanics is defined as the mechanical aspect of movement and posture, including the forces exerted by muscles and gravity on the skeletal structure. Basically, biomechanics (bio (body) mechanics (movement)) is the analysis of how we move. When patients arrive at my clinic, or any clinic with a physical therapist, that PT should assess how the patient moves from the first time they set eyes on them. This information helps the PT begin to formulate a treatment plan.

I injured my knee in the now infamous (in my mind) polka debacle. My medial collateral ligament (MCL) on the inside part of my knee became loose or lax. This ligament and others help my knee stay stable when I walk. But what happens at my knee also impacts what happens at my foot. This is not unique to the knee. What happens at one joint in the body will affect other joints in the body, as well. For example, if there is an injury or restriction in the hip, it can affect how the knee and foot move. If there's an injury or restriction in the shoulder, it can affect how the elbow and hand move. And if there is an injury or restriction in the neck or back, this can affect how the rest of the spine, the pelvis, and even the extremities move.

It's All Connected

Remember that song, "The hip bone's connected to the leg bone. And the leg bone's connected to the foot bone . . ." That is what I'm talking about. It's all connected. Change one thing about the way a joint and muscle move, and it's going to affect something else up or down the chain.

In my case, the knee injury ultimately affected my walking, and changed the biomechanics of my hip and foot, which then, in turn, caused the symptoms of plantar fasciitis. You might need some caffeine for this part unless you are a nerd like me about how the body moves.

The biomechanics of the knee during walking involve complex interactions between bones, muscles, and ligaments to enable movement and to provide stability. Who knew?

Walking can be analyzed through two main types of kinetic chain activities: open chain and closed chain. An open chain activity is where the foot is not in contact with the ground and can move freely (e.g., when you lift your leg off the ground to take a step forward), while a closed chain activity involves the foot being in contact with the ground, and movement occurs with the foot stationary relative to the ground. This starts when your heel hits the ground after you swing it forward when you are walking.

After I injured the ligament that sits on the inside part of my knee, called the medial collateral ligament (MCL), when I swing my leg forward, my knee can feel loose at times. This means it isn't fully stable, because typically when you move your leg, if all is well, you won't even have a sense of how your knee or any other part of your leg feels.

To be clear, I can still walk with my MCL being a little loose. My quadriceps muscle helps me kick my knee out when I walk, so the knee still moves the right way. It just doesn't feel the same as the other knee when I straighten it out. But there's no pain, just a feeling of instability. That small compensation when I kick my leg forward in walking changes my biomechanics just slightly at the knee. But the bigger problem happens when my foot hits the ground.

Unfortunately, when ligaments heal, their fibers don't tighten up again to provide the same stability or support they provided before the injury. The ligament ends up being loose instead of taut. This laxity makes it very important for the muscles around the joint to be as strong as possible to make up for the slack in my ligament, *and* my foot must be in a good position when it hits the floor as I am walking.

Here is a breakdown of what is happening as my foot strikes the ground when walking after the injury:

- My loose MCL (medial collateral ligament) forces my knee into a valgus position, i.e., pushing the knee inward slightly.
- This less-than-advantageous position makes the muscles in my knee and hip work harder to control the movement of the knee joint to keep me moving forward and stop my knee from buckling.
- Because my knee turns in, my foot has to adjust resulting in my arch falling in when I bear weight over that leg.
- The arch falling in contributes to rotational forces on my knee that are more than usual. This puts more force on the injured ligament and the structures around it.
- To complicate things a bit more, my hip muscles were weak and tight, so my knee and foot had to compensate for the decrease in hip stability and flexibility.
- All of this inward force on my foot and arch from the unstable knee and weak, tight hip muscles caused excessive strain on my arch and, as a result, the plantar fascia.
- This causes the fascia to play 'tug of war" with my heel.
- Viola! Plantar fasciitis, heel pain and potentially bone spurs develop.

Evaluating the joints above and below the place of pain is extremely important to see what biomechanics from another joint may be perpetuating or causing pain where you actually feel it.

If I am honest, when I reflect back, I know I noticed some changes in my heel before it started to hurt a great deal. But just like my patients, I did not pay attention to it until it started to affect my day-to-day life.

The answer to my plantar fasciitis, because I caught it early, was to improve the flexibility in my hip and calf. In addition, I had to strengthen the muscles in my hip and knee. And finally, I made adjustments to the inserts in my shoes, called orthotics, and used our SoftWave device. Within two weeks, the pain in my heel was gone. This is the perfect example of how localized pain (heel pain) caused by a change in the biomechanics of my knee, allowed me to discover the tightness in my hip and calf. This tightness was there before the plantar fasciitis and was not an issue *until* I had the knee injury; then that tightness and weakness became a bigger problem and needed to be addressed secondary to the compensatory pattern described above, thus removing the trigger of the continued irritation and allowing the plantar fasciitis to heal.

How Therapy Should Work

You may have also experienced something like this if you went to a physical therapist, chiropractor, or trainer who gave you exercises, did soft tissue mobilization, provided orthotics (if necessary), or gave you an adjustment that resulted in pain relief. You addressed the forces that were contributing to your body compensating because of an injury, tightness, or weakness. When this compensation was addressed, the pain went away. Your body was able to heal, and the pain was relieved. It's really quite remarkable when you think about it. The body can heal itself when we remove the trigger(s) and give it what it needs. But unfortunately, many don't experience a comprehensive program including evaluation of the joints above and below the injury, biomechanics assessment, Softwave, manual therapy, and functional exercise. At the time of this writing, patients are typically only experiencing exercise, and very little, if any, hands-on therapy; except adjustments if you see a chiropractor. Seldom do practitioners spend time with patients to determine the underlying root cause. Symptom management has become too common in many cases. But my hope with The Pain-Free Formula is that you begin to understand what is missing from previous treatment and find the kind of program that will get you better faster.

Tackling The Trigger(s)

In a comprehensive evaluation and assessment, the trigger causing the inflammation may be localized only to the area that was hurting (excess stress on my plantar fascia), but other triggers like my now 'loose' knee ligament and my tight and weak hip contributed to the pain, as well. While this situation wasn't measurable in the sense that we could do a blood test and get a result that showed what the problem was, a trained professional who understands biomechanics can watch you move and spot the potential problems that need to be addressed in order to remove the triggers or stressors and allow the body's innate healing mechanism to take over.

You might recall my analogy from earlier: if you scratch your hand, it becomes painful, red, and puffy. That scratch is the trigger. If the trigger is removed, it's highly likely, if you are generally healthy, that the skin that was injured from the scratch will heal itself without you having to do anything. But if the trigger did not go away, i.e., I kept scratching my hand, the chance of it healing would be greatly reduced. If the inflammation is only localized to the one area, find the tangible trigger(s) and remove them, and the inflammation and pain will often go away. With appropriate exercises, modalities like SoftWave, hands-on treatment, and in my case, support to correct the biomechanics of my foot via orthotics, the pain and inflammation should stay away unless another injury or trigger occurs.

Steps to Eliminate a Biomechanical Tangible Trigger

Find a specialist who has a keen eye for the biomechanics of the body. They should:

- Assess your biomechanics through specialized tests and careful observation of your movements.
- Prescribe exercises that improve flexibility, strength, and joint stabilization—even for joints that aren't directly painful.
- Demonstrate a deep understanding of the joint structures involved, including the capsule, tendons, ligaments, fascia, and nerves.

Other techniques that help my patients heal their bodies from muscle and joint pain that is localized/tangible could include the following:

- Soft Tissue Mobilization: a manual therapy using a type of therapeutic massage to improve function and reduce pain.
- Chiropractic adjustments
- Muscle energy techniques by physical therapists
- Ice or heat: See our blog post: https://newyouhealthandwellness.com/should-i-use-ice-or-heat-joint-pain/
- Appropriate footwear and orthotics
- Taping can support and stabilize joints, muscles, fascia, and ligaments, potentially reducing pain and inflammation.

- Modalities: Several modalities and techniques can be utilized to address joint and muscle pain. If you have seen a physical therapist, you may have had ultrasound, electrical stimulation, TENS units, dry needling, or cupping. You will read about SoftWave, an electrohydraulic shockwave device in the next chapter. This modality has been a game-changer for my patients.
- Acupuncture

All of these techniques can have benefits, especially when performed by a skilled practitioner. Explaining these modalities and treatment strategies goes beyond the scope of this book, but I will talk about many of them on my *Pain-Free Podcast* over time. Please go to https://newyouhealthandwellness.com/the-pain-free-formula-podcast/

This is how I have practiced for decades. Find the trigger, remove the trigger, address the biomechanics, and provide hands-on therapy and functional exercise, and more times than not my patients improved. But recently, one modality has helped me determine whether a patient's pain is localized/tangible or intangible/systemic and has helped patients get long-term relief consistently faster than I have seen in my decades of practice. I mentioned this modality above. It's called SoftWave and you are about to learn how it is helps people with pain.

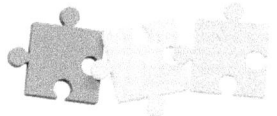

Key Pieces

Movement Affects Pain: Changes in your movement, called compensation, often due to injury, can lead to patterns that cause pain in the area injured but also in other areas. The problem may not be where the pain is. You may have moved a certain way for decades without any problem, but after an injury, inefficient movement patterns can be a barrier to tissue healing.

Biomechanics Matter: Understanding and addressing your body's biomechanics (how you move) is crucial for resolving pain, as poor biomechanics at one joint or muscle can affect others in the body.

Localized Pain Triggers: Identifying and eliminating tangible triggers caused by localized triggers like muscle tightness, joint instability, or improper footwear can help the body heal and alleviate pain.

Find Skilled Practitioners: Techniques like soft tissue mobilization, effective modalities, manual therapy, and proper footwear can be effective in treating localized pain, particularly when applied by skilled practitioners.

Proactive Treatment: Early intervention and addressing the root cause of biomechanical issues can prevent the progression of pain and facilitate quicker recovery.

CHAPTER 7

SoftWave
The Most Effective Modality to Get Rid of Localized Pain

Say Goodbye To Pain One SoftWave At A Time

My right index finger tapped the red button on my phone screen, and the back of my left hand with phone attached fell to the front of my thigh. I took a deep breath and leaned forward to lift myself off my couch and exhaled. Laura, my sister-friend of forty years, had just called to let me know she was five minutes away so I could meet her downstairs in front of my apartment.

The original hardwood floors in this 1923 apartment building creaked under my feet as I slowly walked toward the door. I already regretted agreeing to go with her. I was sure I knew what the outcome was going to be, but I also did not want her to go alone. I felt someone needed to be there as an objective voice of reason. After all, the person she was dragging me to see was about to give his best sales pitch—promising an expensive package of what I thought at the time would be snake oil treatments guaranteed to take her pain away. As a physical therapist for over three decades, and now a master's prepared nurse, I thought I had heard and seen it all. Lofty promises would come that "guaranteed" results only if you met the 1,000-point criteria they listed. Or shiny gadgets that whirred with high-tech sounding bells and whistles would be on display, only to spew out useless reports that did not provide anything close to the value that they were portrayed as having on the Instagram or Facebook ad.

My apartment door clicked shut, and the keys in my hand jingled as I shimmied them from the lock and slid them into my coat pocket. My hand glided down the cool wooden handrail, and I rounded the corner to descend the additional creaky stairs. As I turned the deadbolt at the bottom of the stairs, the zipper on the sleeve of my three-quarter-length coat clanged against the knob of the last outside door. And when I pulled it open, a gush of cool autumn air filled my lungs.

Ding!

I rustled my phone from my pocket and read the text. "I'm here."

Securing my door behind me, I walked up toward the white SUV, crouched a little, and waved at Laura sitting in the driver's seat. I yanked the car door open and hopped in. "Perfect timing," I said as I smiled, trying to hide my slight irritation about the trip we were about to take. "Thanks again for coming with me," she said. "I want your expert opinion."

"Of course, no problem." I paused. "But I already gave you my expert opinion. Remember?"

Laura pulled out from in front of my building and started to drive. "Yeah, after you looked at the website for like a millisecond," she quipped.

She was right. A week prior, I had pulled up the website related to the device we were about to witness and spent probably less than a minute looking through the information. Silence filled the car.

"This guy said he has used this on tons of people, and they all get better."

I turned my head to look out the passenger window.

"You are rolling your eyes, aren't you," she groaned.

"No," I lied. She knew me too well. My gaze turned toward her. "Seriously, the thing looks like a space-age ultrasound machine," I finally said.

"I can't see how this is going to help your shoulder. All these machines are the same."

"Really?" I could hear her enthusiasm deflate. "You've seen it before?"

"Well, no. I haven't seen *that* exact machine." I paused. "But remember, I have been in this business forever and I have looked at so many of these 'new' machines over the years. I've sat through countless presentations in the clinic by medical device reps. I am not embarrassed to say I showed up primarily to get a free lunch. Over decades of listening to these salespeople and trying their devices, I have never seen anything that helped my patients more than what I already did manually, along with exercise, and through education.

Physical therapists (PTs) are a different breed when it comes to using modalities. At least I was, and so are many of the other PTs I grew up in the ranks with. I considered myself old school because I still actually put my hands on my patients to help them address their muscle and joint issues. Manual therapy, seemingly a lost art among some of the younger generation of physical therapists, had always set us apart from other professionals. Our evaluations were thorough, and in orthopedics and pelvic health, treatments consisted of mobilizing muscle tissue and joints, optimizing biomechanics, and working with the fascia and other tissues in the body to gain freer, more comfortable movements. Before insurance started paying less and less for each visit, we actually spent quality time with our patients to determine how we could create the best outcomes for them. We did not rely on gadgets and expensive machines because we did not have to. Our patients often got better when our interventions helped them move more efficiently and when we explained to them what was contributing to their pain so they could eliminate those triggers.

"This one is supposed to be different," Laura piped in.

"What's it called again?" I asked as I squinted at my phone screen and searched for a name on the website.

"SoftWave therapy," Laura answered.

SoftWave Trial

As we got closer to the house, Laura reminded me that the person who had the device was kind enough to bring it to our friend's house so she could try it on her shoulder. Fully recognizing the stern warning that she was giving me, because I gave the same type of speech to my son as he was growing up when he had to accompany his dad and me to some gathering he did not want to be at, I responded.

"Okay, I am fine. This will be fun."

Now, she rolled her eyes.

The drive was about twenty minutes and dusk was settling in. The trees in Wisconsin were turning their vibrant colors for the fall season.

Laura asked, "Oh, hey, did you get the studies that I sent you from the guy?"

"Yeah, I did."

"Did you look at them?"

"I will." I continued. "Now remember what I said. Don't be disappointed if this doesn't do what he says it's going to do."

"Man, I have never heard you be so negative."

"I'm not being negative," I hesitated. "Just realistic."

"Can you just have an open mind? I want to try this on my shoulder. It's supposed to be amazing, and you know I have tried everything."

"Yes. I know." My stomach panged a little, thinking back to the fact that I wasn't only her friend, I was the physical therapist who had worked on her shoulder. "We did get you to be pain-free for almost everything that you do."

"That's true, but it still hurts when I lift it way over my head or if I sleep that way I told you about."

I gave her the side eye. And we got out of the car. We had reached our destination.

"Yeah," she responded as both our car doors slammed shut. "I know I am not supposed to sleep with my arm that way." She shrugged as we walked up the sidewalk to the house. "But I can't help it. It just happens."

As Laura reached out to knock on the door of our friend Sue's house, I heard her whisper, "Be nice."

"I am always nice," I replied with a grin.

To our surprise, a man wearing a red plaid flannel who was not my friend's husband opened the door and boomed, "Well, hello!"

"Hey Dave," Laura answered. She proceeded forward and passed by the six-foot-tall stranger as he held the outside screen door open.

"Thanks," I said, smiling as I walked past him, sideways, into the house.

"You must be Stacey," I heard him say behind me.

I turned toward him behind me and walked backward. "It's nice to meet you."

I stopped and our elbows met, as this was the fall of 2020, and most people either avoided any contact at all or gave the habitual elbow tap.

Our friend Sue, who was also a physical therapist, offered her home to use for this demonstration. We all stood around and small talk ensued. Sue set out some healthy snacks, as usual.

After the pleasantries slowed, Dave motioned Laura over to the hot seat: a stool from the kitchen counter that sat next to the machine that I had seen on the website.

"This is SoftWave," Dave explained as he motioned toward the device. He then began giving his spiel about what it did.

I was more interested in the delicious dip that Sue had put out, so I dunked my celery stick deep into the bowl to get a big scoop and then sat back in the wooden chair next to the host getting settled in for the demonstration. "I feel like we are at a multilevel marketing meeting," I whispered to Sue. She and I tried to stifle a laugh.

It took everything I had in my power not to slink down in the chair with my arms crossed over my chest, completely closing my body language off to our presenter and his magic machine. Instead, I leaned forward, elbows on the table, not so quietly chewing my celery and listened as he briefly explained what this device, from a company called SoftWave TRT, could do.

I could feel Sue's skepticism emanating from the chair next to me. I did not want to look her way because I was afraid we would end up experiencing a bout of that uncontrollable laughter that only ever happens between besties at the most inopportune time.

Dave called it an electrohydraulic shockwave device, which at the time meant nothing to me except that maybe it involved water and electricity. *That's* a great combination, I thought. The machine started to whir a bit, and as he touched a button on the hose-like structure that came out of the device, a few sparks of light and loud clicks emanated out of its dome-like membrane.

Sue and I jumped a little in our seats. Our eyes met for a second, and I heard her say, "Cool."

I cleared my throat, and hated to admit this, but it did look pretty cool. It reminded me of something I would have seen on *Star Trek*.

Laura rolled her t-shirt up to expose her shoulder and Dave was about to start the treatment. As Dave set the applicator on her skin, I could see Laura tense up a bit and her eyes open wider, so I blurted out, "Wait, does that hurt?" My instinct was to protect my friend.

Dave paused and held the applicator up in midair. "It's not really painful," he responded. "It'll be a bit sensitive in some areas where there is inflammation, but that goes away."

He was ready to start again.

"So, what's it doing though?" I asked. "Does it tell you where the inflammation is?"

"Kind of," he answered. "Laura will tell me where she feels it and that is likely where the inflammation is. And as the inflammation decreases, she will feel it less and less."

"Really? What will she feel everywhere else?" Sue asked.

"Not much. Just a bit of tapping."

"Interesting," I said, throwing a slow glance at Sue with eyebrows lifted.

I found myself leaning back in my chair again.

"Laura, first, before we start, does your shoulder hurt right now?"

Her arms were resting naturally at her side. "No," she answered.

"Can you show me what you are doing when it does hurt?" Dave asked.

Laura raised her arm up over her head. It was a motion I had seen her do a hundred times before in therapy. When I first saw her in the clinic, she could barely lift her arm. But after six weeks of PT twice a week, we got her to the point where she was at that moment and that lasted for a good six months.

"It only hurts when I get up to here." She raised her arm way up over her head, grimacing at the very end of the motion. "And if I lay on it like that, it ends up waking me up." I could tell she was avoiding looking at me.

"Okay, thanks. That will be a good test for us at the end of the treatment."

I was slightly impressed. Asking a patient to perform the motion that hurts prior to treatment is good practice, so that they can repeat the motion after the treatment to assess its effectiveness. *Half a gold star for Dave*, I thought.

With the applicator in hand and its hose over his shoulder, Dave asked. "Ready?"

"Yep," she said, and her lips tightened a bit.

Dave proceeded to put the squishy (my most specific medical term) dome full of water at the end of the applicator against Laura's shoulder. He put a bit of pressure on it to flatten it out. Sue and I inched forward a bit in our seats.

He pressed the button and the sparks flashed. All three of us jumped again a bit. The clicking continued, and as he pressed the dome further against her skin, the flashes of light disappeared and then reappeared in sequence with the clicks as he was running the applicator head slowly around her shoulder.

"How does it feel?" he asked above audible clicking sound as he moved the applicator around.

She responded, "I only feel that tapping."

But seconds later, she said, "Okay, wait. Right there."

Dave stopped the movement of the applicator, but let the pulses keep going as he hovered over the painful area. "I can feel it going deeper into my shoulder, right there," Laura stated. "That's usually where I get my pain."

I looked at Sue. "Huh," I whispered.

Sue and I knew that was way more than just a little interesting. While Laura's arm was resting at her side, a position that didn't normally cause pain, the applicator was now over thespot where Laura had experienced pain, both past and present. In fact, it was in the exact spot that she had pain when she raised her arm over her head. Dave did not tell her it was going to hurt there. She offered that information up herself.

Remember, Laura only ever had pain when she raised her arm. However, while the machine was whirring and steadily treating that area, Laura felt a discomfort or a sensation over the exact spot that she had calcific tendonitis. Sue and I looked at each other as if we were thinking the same thing. *How in the world did the device pick up on the calcified area in her biceps tendon without her moving?* I'd never seen anything like that.

"Hmm," I heard myself mutter again.

The treatment, consisting of the clicking and synchronized flashes of light were a result of sparks from an electrode inside the applicator, continued for approximately eight to ten minutes. During this time, Laura reported less pain each and every time Dave had moved the probe over the area that was the issue. When the pain was nearly gone, Dave pushed the button on the probe and the clicking stopped.

"Okay, that's it," he said.

"That's it?" Laura asked.

"Yep, that's it." He smiled.

"That wasn't bad at all," Laura said, as she sat up a little taller in her seat.

"What did it feel like?" Sue asked.

"It's so weird. It just feels like tapping until he went over that spot in the front of my shoulder, and then it was kind of stingy there. It did not really hurt. But each time he came back to it, it stung less, until eventually, it was practically gone."

"Hmm." At this point, it was all I seemed to be able to say.

"Okay," Dave said, "lift your arm up."

Laura lifted her arm exactly the way she had done approximately ten minutes earlier. She was silent for a second, brought her arm back down to her side and quickly lifted it again. This time, she lifted it higher and behind her body.

"Holy crap," she said. "It doesn't hurt. The pain is gone."

Is This For Real?

That experience with Laura, my sister from another mister, led me on an incredible path of discovery. I was absolutely convinced that Laura's experience, that is, her pain relief, was not going to last. I even remember saying to her on the ride home, "Don't get your hopes up, it's probably going to hurt again in the next couple of days."

But it did not.

After having the one SoftWave treatment, she literally went without pain until she injured herself playing pickleball two years later!

After seeing this result, to say I was intrigued would be an understatement. I hadn't seen anything like this in my decades of practice. Accompanied by a healthy dose of skepticism, I started digging into the research. I had extra time, as this was during Covid, and my analytical brain searched and searched to see if I could explain this away as a fluke. Instead, I found solid research supporting the use of shockwave for pain relief. Over time, I tried many different devices, even devices called radial pressure wave that say they are shockwave, but they are not. I came back to SoftWave because it was the most comfortable and had excellent outcomes in the research. I had to take a bit of a leap of faith since insurance did not cover it.

Why doesn't insurance cover it? My best guess is that due to all the devices on the market, and the varying outcomes with the devices that aren't true shockwave (and even with those that are), protocols are inconsistent, and so are results. That is a problem that the shockwave industry has to solve. I could have waited for insurance coverage, which could be years away (or never), but I wanted to bring this accelerated healing experience to patients in my community. Having now been exposed to the results of this, I felt it was unethical if I did not. So, though no one in the area had SoftWave, I opened my own clinic, starting from scratch, during Covid, while I was in my full-time program earning my master's degree in nursing. It was a wild ride, but that is a story for another time.

Truth be told, my patients who receive SoftWave therapy at my clinic do not usually have a 'one and done' encounter like Laura. If done correctly, and if the issue is localized to the area I am treating, it usually takes three weekly treatments to have a 50 to 100 percent reduction in pain. And some need six treatments in total. There have been a few single treatments resulting in complete pain relief since I started treating with SoftWave, but most need more work on their biomechanics, strength, and flexibility. If the inflammation is systemic (we will talk about that in upcoming chapters), I work with the patient on finding and removing the intangible triggers that we discover to achieve complete relief. Three to six treatments of SoftWave, however, are usually the most my patients need for resolution of the pain if the inflammation is only localized. That is a far cry from the ten to fifteen treatments my patients would previously need, on average, for significant or complete relief in traditional physical therapy.

It's still unbelievable to me, but SoftWave is now one of the most important tools in my toolbox. Prior to utilizing SoftWave, I truly never saw any other modality work as consistently and as successfully as SoftWave does. I still use manual therapy, including soft tissue mobilization and muscle energy techniques, as well as exercise, but SoftWave treatment makes all of the treatments I do more effective and less painful for my patients.

There's a reason I have a sign in my office that says, "Maybe swearing will help." Prior to SoftWave, it wasn't unusual for me to dig my thumbs, knuckles, and occasionally an elbow into trigger points (a hyperirritable spot in a muscle) to release it and eventually result in significant relief for my patients. But trigger point therapy as well as dry needling and other therapies can, at times, be a long process to get sustained relief, and it's quite uncomfortable.

But now SoftWave, an electrohydraulic, broadly focused shockwave device, primes the area I am working on. It allows me to get much deeper, much faster after it's applied, and this allows for less discomfort and accelerated healing when I do my hands-on manual therapy, muscle energy adjustments, or mobilization of joints. One of my patients, Cindy, a massage therapist of twenty years, describes SoftWave as a two-hour massage in ten minutes. Others describe it as a miracle. One patient asked, "Is it bad that I start dreaming about my SoftWave appointment a few days before I see you?"

Most of my patients, like me, had never experienced a treatment where, after one visit, they can walk out of my office pain-free for the first time in weeks, months, and even years. Calling SoftWave a miracle may be a stretch, but it is definitely a game-changer.

Where's the Research?

If you are a healthcare provider, researcher, or just a highly motivated educated consumer who wants to do whatever they can for their health to improve their chances of living a long, active life, you will want to see the research. If you are skeptical, that's good! As you have read, so was I.

I honestly believe there was divine intervention regarding my witnessing Laura's experience. I wouldn't have believed it if I hadn't been there. And I wouldn't have necessarily believed she had that much improvement if I hadn't known and trusted her basically my whole life. But even after seeing the dramatic effect for Laura, I wasn't ready to jump into the SoftWave camp just yet. After all, in my experience, she represented patient zero. But would there be more who experienced improvement? Or was that just a fluke? I was experienced enough to know that a result like hers was likely rare, but nonetheless it intrigued me, so I was very motivated to learn more. As my healthy dose of skepticism slowly morphed into extreme curiosity, I dove into the shockwave research.

After much digging, research revealed there are three different types of true shockwave devices on the market. And as I read the research, I saw that the outcomes differed significantly for each of the devices. Some research showed how amazing shockwave was, and others showed it was just the same as other modalities. This was a common occurrence. It was very confusing.

The answer could only be a result of three things:

- What I witnessed with Laura was a fluke
- The studies were poorly designed

- All the devices were not the same, meaning not every shockwave device had the same effects

I learned that the latter (not every shockwave device was the same) was a big part of the discrepancies in the research. And even more interesting, there is a device referred to as shockwave that, as it turns out, does *not* produce a shockwave at all.

The research is vast and often very confusing. More on that later. But I was intrigued and determined to learn.

Three Types of True Shockwave

Here's what more in-depth digging revealed:

The three types of TRUE shockwave devices (that actually produce a genuine shockwave) are sold as low-intensity devices. And like any medical device company, each of them says that theirs is the best, and they have opinions, and some but not all have a few research studies sprinkled in to show why their device is better than the others. But I wasn't interested in opinions; I wanted to find the facts. So, I plowed through countless full-text resources about shockwave therapy related to orthopedics, pelvic health, sexual health, and more. I did not just read through the abstracts (a general synopsis) or the conclusions. Nope, I painstakingly read through all the different parts of the research studies, i.e., the abstract, the introduction, the materials and methods, the statistics and results, the discussions, and the conclusions. Normally, I wouldn't have the time to do such an in-depth analysis, but the Covid shutdown provided me with extra time, and this journey was definitely more exciting than another Zoom call about new recipes I could make. I wanted to know how and why it worked so differently than anything I had ever seen before, and why there were so many different protocols about how to use the devices and so many different outcomes.

As I was doing the research, I was also starting my nursing program, and at that point, most of my program was online as my clinicals hadn't started yet, so I could work anywhere. Many people were not traveling at that time yet, but with mask on, I sought out any shockwave device I could find to try them out. I even tried the device that says it is a shockwave-type product, but it doesn't even produce a shockwave. And the results were, in my opinion, astonishing.

The Results Were In

As mentioned, there are three types of true shockwave devices:

1. Electrohydraulic (SoftWave is this type of device)
2. Electromagnetic
3. Piezoelectric

All of these true shockwave devices can help to address inflammation, and as a result, decrease pain and, in some cases, accelerate healing. But you'll see in a moment why SoftWave is, in my opinion and in my patients' experience, a cut above the rest. People who have other devices usually say shockwave devices are all the same, but I definitely did not have the same experience with the other devices that I did with SoftWave. Before we go into how true shockwave works, I would be remiss if I did not explain something to you first.

Not All Shockwave is TRUE Shockwave

Somewhere in the past, when shockwave devices were coming on the market, the International Society for Medical Shockwave Therapy (ISMST) allowed medical devices called radial pressure waves to be a part of the discussion about shockwave. Even though, technically, radial devices do not produce shockwaves, they were described as such.

142   THE PAIN FREE FORMULA

I mention this here because in much of the research and in clinics around the US, radial devices are still described as shockwave. Practitioners who purchased these radial devices still believe they have devices that produce shockwaves. I know because they enroll in my Shockwave courses and get annoyed with me when I share the facts of physics with the group. The physics clearly shows that radial devices do not produce shockwaves.

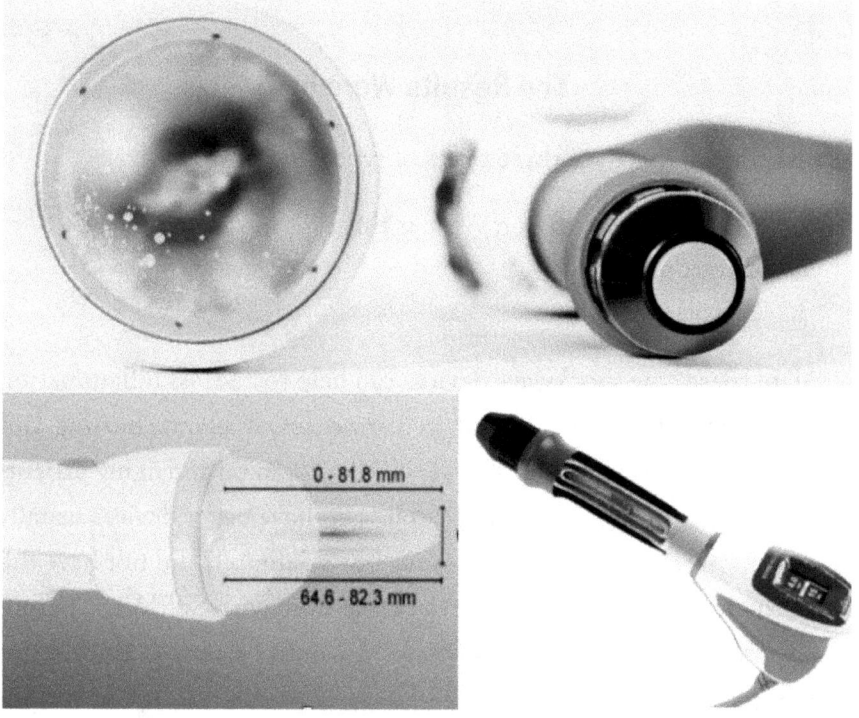

Figure 7.1 There are differences between the radial device on the right (doesn't create a shockwave) and the SoftWave device on the left (an electrohydraulic broad -ocused true shockwave device).

SOFTWAVE 143

Figure 7.1 depicts what SoftWave's true shockwave applicator looks like versus a radial pressure wave device.

Radial devices produce pressure waves from compressed air, which act like a jackhammer smacking against the tissues. See Figure 7.2. It creates significant microtrauma, soreness, and sometimes bruising and swelling. If your practitioner tells you that you are going to feel significant pain and soreness for two to three weeks, and then you will start to feel better, nine times out of ten, they have a radial device, not a true shockwave device. I have tried this device on heel and hand pain, and it was very painful.

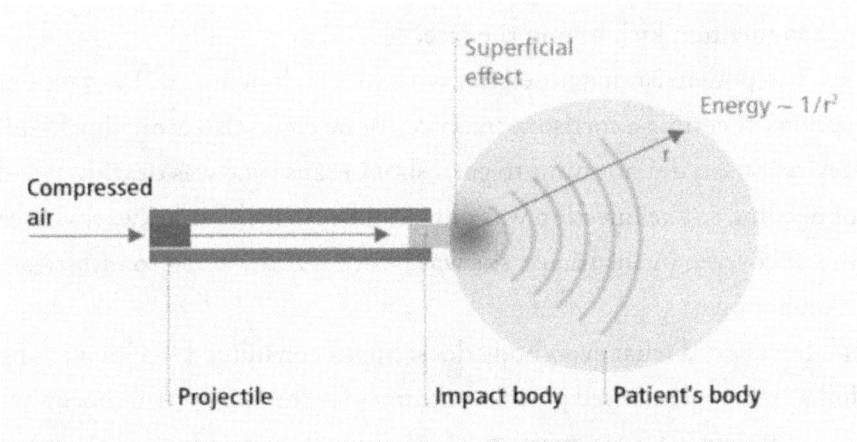

Figure 7.2 An example of a radial device and its impact on the body. The biological effect starts to weaken after penetrating 5 or 6 mm into the skin, whereas SoftWave devices can have a biological effect up to 12 cm into the body.

Ask Susan

Don't take my word for it. Susan's experience is a typical example of what I hear about the use of radial pressure waves. This story isn't here to infer radial wave devices are inferior or superior to true shockwave.

But I believe it's important that anyone looking for a service that can help them should be given accurate information about the technology, and, whenever possible, the experience they are expected to have.

Susan developed excruciating pain in the ball of her foot. It hurt as soon as she put any weight on her leg when she got out of bed in the morning but worsened later as the day progressed. Each day, when it was irritated, she would put most of her weight on her right foot and limp her way to wherever she was going. This went on for a few months before she finally went to see a podiatrist. At the evaluation, he stuck his finger in between her second and third metatarsals, the bones in the ball of the foot. Like most people with pain there, she wanted to scream, not to mention kick him in the face.

The podiatrist diagnosed her with Morton's neuroma. He gave her options of getting a cortisone injection, or he could also use a "shockwave" device. Susan did not want to get a shot because she was deathly afraid of needles, so the injection was out. And because the shockwave device wasn't covered by insurance, she was hesitant and wanted to investigate it on her own.

So, she did what everybody does: Susan consulted Dr. Google. The links on Google showed positive outcomes for the search term 'shockwave and foot pain.' The vast majority of information referred to radial devices, not true shockwave devices. But Susan did not know the difference. Why would she? The first time she ever heard the term "shockwave" was at her podiatrist's office just a day or so prior. And now Google confirmed it worked, so it must be true.

Susan called the podiatrist's office a few days later and made an appointment, hoping to get rid of the pain in her foot without having to get an injection.

Fast forward a few years, and Susan had come to my office for the SoftWave trial that we offer for our potential patients. She fidgeted in her seat a bit when she sat down. I asked her where she heard about us, and she replied that she saw one of my appearances on a local television show called *The Morning Blend*. "The lady on the show said it worked for her, so I thought I would give it a try."

I smiled. I had appeared on *The Morning Blend* several times with patients who had come to our clinic. This was a great way to show prospective patients what the experience was like from people who had actually felt the treatment. I started asking Susan questions based on her answers from the health questionnaire that she filled in before the appointment.

"I see you have had foot pain before," I confirmed.

"Yes, but on the other foot," Susan replied.

"Okay, how long ago was that?" I asked.

"About three years ago."

"Does that foot bother you anymore?"

"Not too much. Here and there."

"And your right foot? How was it walking in here today?"

"Horrible. I can barely walk by this time of day."

"I know that it is a terrible feeling. It's definitely a typical symptom of Morton's neuroma." I paused and read through some of her information before asking, "What did you do for the other foot?"

"I had some shockwave therapy," Susan replied.

I glanced at her curiously above the glasses that sat low on the bridge of my nose. "You had shockwave therapy?" Knowing that most patients in my area at that time had never seen SoftWave before, and I was the only person in my town at that time who had a machine, I asked her, "What was that experience like?"

"It hurt like hell," she replied.

"But it helped?" I asked.

"Well, it never completely went away. But it is definitely a whole lot better. And I suppose I could have gone in for more treatments, but I could only stand having three. It was so painful I did not want to go back.

But it did get better after about three or four weeks of limping around."

Right then and there, I knew she had treatment with a radial device, not a true shockwave device.

"I'm surprised that you came to see me then."

"Yeah, well, I wasn't sure, and to be honest," she shifted in her chair, "I was a little worried this is going to hurt the same as last time. But when I watched the video again, it looked different than what I had a couple years ago, and Molly, the lady on the show, said it did not really hurt and that it got rid of pain that she was having for a long time."

Susan's story illustrates the significant difference between radial pressure wave therapy and SoftWave therapy. Radial pressure wave can be effective for superficial tissue, but patients report the treatment hurts significantly more than SoftWave. And others I have talked to who have experienced radial devices for diagnosis like tendonitis or bursitis concur with Susan. They struggle with whether to finish the treatment plan because of how painful the treatment is. Radial devices can work for these superficial injuries, but for some it can be a very agonizing process.

On the other hand, I use SoftWave on all muscles and joints in the body, including to treat sensitive areas like the pelvic floor for diagnosis such as vulvodynia, dyspareunia (painful intercourse), and pelvic pain in men and women. And with SoftWave therapy, the vast majority of my patients walk out of their first treatment with no pain or significantly less pain. Susan was over the moon after her first treatment. She walked out with her right foot feeling better than the left foot that she had treated years earlier. Upon completion of four visits which included SoftWave, specific exercises based on a biomechanical analysis, some shoe wear suggestions, and a couple bits of homework to do at home, Susan was completely pain-free and walking on trails in Arizona, something she wouldn't have considered doing a few months before.

How can you tell if a clinic has a radial device and they are calling it shockwave?

I'll be honest, it's not easy. Many times, the clinician who has a radial device will be adamant that it is a shockwave device. They can even show you studies that are titled extracorporeal shockwave therapy (ESWT), but the study is actually using a radial device, not a true shockwave device. Talk about confusing! Some researchers in the past and some in the present still aren't getting it right.

ESWT is meant to be descriptive of all shockwave therapy, but unfortunately along the way, radial devices, which as you now know do not produce shockwaves, snuck under the umbrella of ESWT. As I searched for the answer as to why, it appears that true shockwave devices produce a radial wave, but radial devices do not produce shockwaves. Someday this distinction may be fixed, but for now, when you are reading a pamphlet from a company saying they have a shockwave device, it's up to you to ask what kind of shockwave the device produces.

When you ask them, and they give you any of the answers below, or you see these words listed on their site or in brochures or pamphlets, then it is a radial device, and you can expect the pain to be worse before it gets better.

If on a company's website, or on any of their materials, it says any of the following:

- RPWT: Radial Pressure Wave Therapy
- rESWT: Radial Extracorporeal Shock Wave Therapy (sometimes used interchangeably with RPWT, though technically not a shockwave)
- R-PWT: Radial-Pulse Wave Therapy
- EPAT: Extracorporeal Pulse-Activated Therapy

Then it's a radial device.

> **PSA:** Now that you know that radial devices aren't shockwave devices from a physics standpoint, it's not a good idea to accuse those clinics of false advertising. I can almost guarantee they were told by whoever sold it to them that they were buying a shockwave device. I am already seeing some large companies start making the distinction between radial devices and shockwave devices on their websites. I am hopeful that this will continue to change and become more accurate as time goes on. Also, please understand that radial devices, although painful, can be effective on superficial injuries, such as tendonitis, bursitis, etc. But they tend to be ineffective for issues that are inside the joint or deep in the muscle or joint. They also can't be used on acute injuries and have other restrictions.

If you don't see any of the acronyms previously listed on the clinic's website or a picture of the applicator, ask them if it hurts and if it's expected to get worse before it gets better. This won't definitively let you know that it is a radial device, but it helps to narrow it down.

How Does SoftWave Differentiate Itself from Other True Shockwave Devices?

Now that you understand what a radial device is, and that besides being painful, it can be beneficial with some of the more superficial issues, this leaves us with the true shockwave devices. If you are like me, you want to choose the best treatment for your situation. Therefore, use this section as a starting point for your own research.

As a reminder, I mentioned there are three different *true* shockwave devices, i.e., devices that actually produce shockwaves.

They are:

Electrohydraulic
Electromagnetic
Piezoelectric

I already mentioned that electrohydraulic devices like SoftWave travel deeper and wider into the tissues than the electromagnetic or piezoelectric products.

The biggest differentiating factor that you will find between SoftWave and the other devices, including other electrohydraulic devices, is the applicator. This is the part of the device shown in Figure 7.1 that actually touches the patient.

Inside of it, there is an electrode that produces a spark, which is the shockwave. This is the "electro" in electrohydraulic. The other aspect of the SoftWave applicator, as you can see below, is the water inside the dome where the electrode sits. This is the hydraulic part. And if that's not enough to hurt your brain, like it did mine when I was learning all this, SoftWave's applicator head is significantly different than *all* the other true shockwave devices. So what? You might ask.

Well, all other true shockwave devices are solely focused, meaning all the energy is focused to one small point (see Figure 7.3), and therefore their treatment zone only targets one certain spot. The focused only device applicator has to move around a lot because it only covers a small treatment zone. In addition, you have to use many more shocks at much higher energies to get similar results to SoftWave's broad focused treatment.

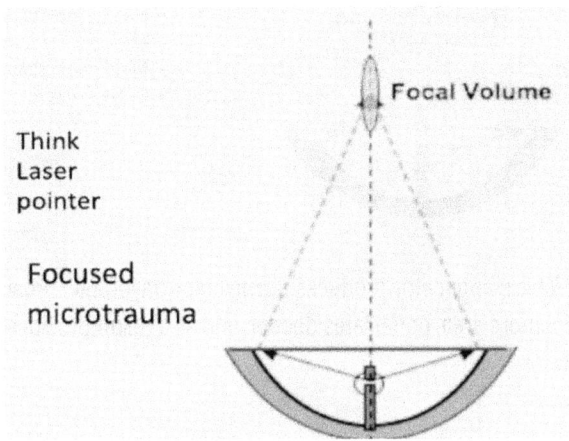

Figure 7.3 Focused-only shockwave devices. Their energy comes out of the applicator like a laser.

Have you seen those videos of cats following the dot shining on the ground from a laser pointer? That's what a solely-focused applicator does; it combines all its energy to that one dot or treatment zone. If you know exactly the spot that you want to treat, whether it be a kidney stone (very high-intensity focused shock waves are used to break up kidney stones in a hospital setting) or a fracture/broken bone, you know exactly where the problem is, and solely-focused shockwave applicators can be good, yet painful, for those diagnoses. But when all the energy is focused on just one spot, it can be very uncomfortable for the patient. Not quite as uncomfortable as a radial device, but definitely uncomfortable. And the treatment time is longer because it will require more shocks to treat an area that is larger than a pinpoint of light.

SoftWave's applicator, by comparison, is broad-focused. It is the only shockwave applicator that has both a wide treatment zone and a focused one. See Figure 7.4.

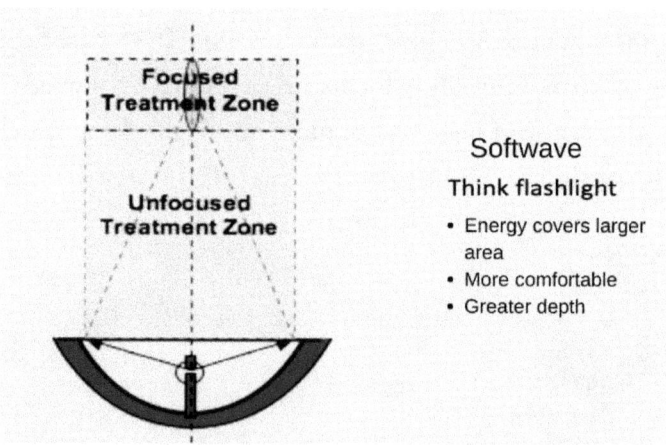

Figure 7.4 SoftWave's applicator produces a true electrohydraulic broad-focused shockwave that covers more area, penetrates deeper, and as a result provides a more comfortable treatment.

This means two things:

1. SoftWave is much more comfortable, even when the energy is turned up.
2. SoftWave can reach both superficial and deeper tissues.

Because SoftWave is so versatile, I can treat superficial issues like tendonitis, bursitis, or deep tissues like joint capsules (think frozen shoulder or adhesive capsulitis), arthritic joint surfaces, the three deep layers of the pelvic floor, and deep layers of the hip and back. And I am not alone. Other practitioners such as Lance Frank PT, DPT, MH, a physical therapist specializing in orthopedics and men's pelvic health, also tried all of the true shockwave devices for his patients.

SoftWave provided the best outcomes at his Flex PT clinic in Atlanta, Georgia. Lance also has a popular TikTok channel where his handle is "Lance_in_your_pants." Definitely check him out.

Lance reports, "I tried all three true shockwave devices and found that SoftWave was the one that gave my patients consistent positive outcomes. The others tended to be hit or miss. Because they were focused only, it was hard to find the right spot and stay on that spot to get the best outcomes."

But How Does It Work?

Now that I have established that I chose SoftWave for my patients due to:

- Its effectiveness
- Its comfort level for my patients
- The fact that it can treat both superficial and very deep structures

How the heck does it actually work?

In Chapter 5, I discussed inflammation and the different phases necessary to result in healing of tissues in the body. With our SoftWave treatment, we have two goals: if there is inflammation, we want to decrease it to the point that it is no longer painful or limiting. If there is muscle tension due to decreased blood flow or inflammation, we want to improve the blood flow (without damaging the tissue) to address the tension and the inflammation, if necessary.

Take my knee, for example. After the beer barrel polka took me out (you read about that story in the introduction) and I found out that my knee was, in fact, full of arthritis that had been there for years, what struck me most after my X-rays was that prior to my injury on the dance floor, I did not have any pain.

Let me say that again,

I had no pain even though there was clearly significant arthritis and inflammation in my knee joint prior to my injury.

During the dancing, I heard a 'pop.' The searing pain that followed was my body's way of telling me, 'ah, something bad just happened.' Whether it was scar tissue tearing, my medial collateral ligament tearing away from the meniscus, or a lightning bolt shooting through me because I hadn't been to church in a while, I will never know. But what I did know from my knee swelling up like a balloon and the preceding pain was that there was a significant amount of new inflammation, and some sort of injury that my body wanted to protect me from until it healed. That is why I couldn't put weight on my leg. The pain was so severe that I could only move around via crutches the morning after the wedding. I couldn't put even a slight amount of weight on my leg without experiencing the feeling of a hot poker slamming through my knee.

But when I applied SoftWave to this injury the next day, the swelling almost immediately went down. And over time, the pain dissipated so that after three treatments (in ten days), I could walk without crutches.

The research shows that when SoftWave is applied to an area where there is inflammation, when applied correctly, the superficial or deep stimulus from the waves that are entering the body and running in between the spaces between the bones in the joint, or deep into the muscle, tell the brain to pay attention to the area being treated. And at the time, molecules that help move inflammation toward healing, such as stem cells, M2 macrophages, and others travel to the area being treated. This results in an anti-inflammatory effect. And as you now know, the anti-inflammatory effect precedes the tissues' ability to fully heal.

If the inflammation is only localized, as in my case from the injury, and not systemic as described in the following chapters, after treatments with SoftWave, the healing process continues. As a result, the inflammation reduces to a point below the pain threshold, or it reduces to no inflammation at all. In my arthritic knee, the inflammation must be under my pain threshold as I no longer have pain, *even though I still have arthritis*. If you did not have significant inflammation in the joint prior to an injury, SoftWave can accelerate the healing process so the tissue can return to normal.

One example of SoftWave working with the body's innate healing process was related to a runner with severe Achilles tendonitis. The middle-aged male had two surgeries on his Achilles tendon due to pain as well as his inability to run and cycle to his liking. This patient's MRI showed significant swelling in his Achilles tendon, as seen in the Figure 7.5 below on the left, indicated by the arrows.

154   THE PAIN FREE FORMULA

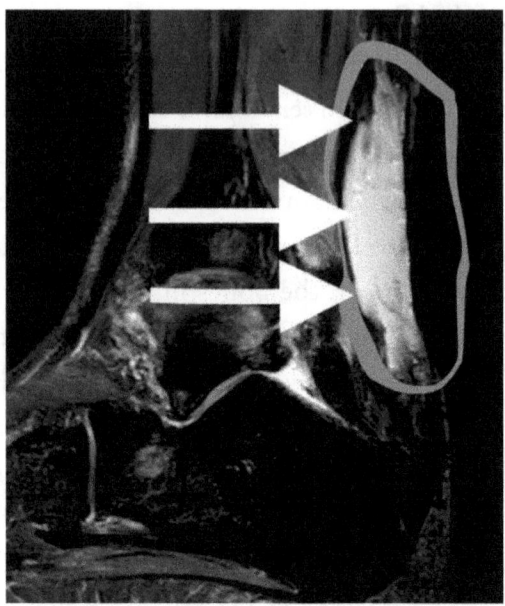

Figure 7.5 Achilles tendonitis and fibrosis prior to Softwave

The patient had five treatments of SoftWave over eight weeks and was able to return to running and cycling. The patient had a follow-up MRI four years later to see the progress, and you can see the difference in Figure 7.6.

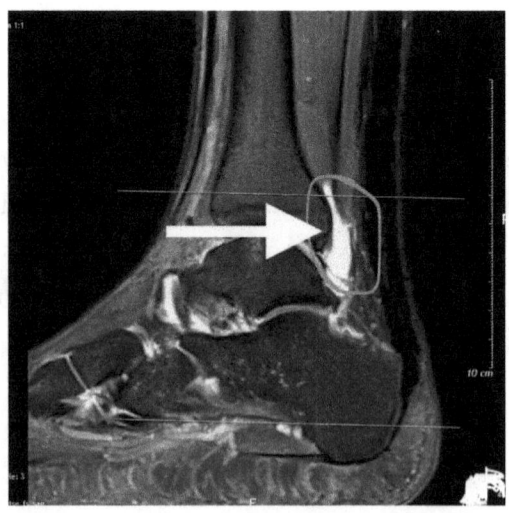

Figure 7.6

Normally, after an injury with scarring or fibrosis developing, it wouldn't get better, especially if the person went back to activities like running. But you can see that there is very little swelling or fibrosis in the area of the Achilles tendon after FOUR years, despite his continued high-impact activity. The body can heal when the triggers of inflammation are taken away and it's given what it needs to heal.

SoftWave's ability to bring blood flow to the area without creating trauma is another aspect that sets it apart from the rest of the shockwave devices. This increased blood flow brings the molecules necessary to address inflammation to the area treated, which can result in decreased pain, but there's a further benefit for another type of tissue.

What About Muscle Pain? "Now That's a Good Hurt."

It makes sense that if inflammation is causing pain, SoftWave would work like a charm, and it does. But what about muscle pain that may or may not be coming from inflammation? Can it help with that?

Yes. It can.

The stimulation that the wave provides to the tissues being treated increases blood flow to the area immediately. Therefore, if a muscle is guarding (holding in a partial state of contraction to protect the injured area), this increased blood flow can relax the muscle immediately and decrease pain. This is what happened to Steve. Steve's muscles went into guarding mode after he hurt his back and created agony whenever he tried to move. Remember, this is the body wanting to help you. Your brain thinks, *If I don't move, I won't hurt myself.* So if you try to move, your brain is sending messages to your muscles to create pain, so you stay put.

In addition to relaxing the muscle, another amazing effect of shockwave is a process called *neoangiogenesis*. This means that new (neo) blood vessels (angio) grow (genesis). This provides more nourishment to what may have become an ischemic muscle, i.e., a muscle that lacks blood flow due to a constant state of partial contraction. Think of your upper trapezius muscles. They connect your neck to your shoulders. When you have a sore 'upper trap,' you grab that area between your head and shoulders instinctively and give it a squeeze. You or someone you allow to press into that area can feel 'knots' or hard areas of the muscle. Some of these knots may be referred to as trigger points by medical professionals.

What causes these trigger points? No one seems to know exactly what causes them, but we do know what we can do to relieve the pain. Press on them. Massage them. Let therapists like me stick their thumbs, knuckles, or even elbows into them. Dry needle them. This initially causes significant discomfort, but when you hold the pressure there, the muscle eventually relents, and the pain can go away.

Tamping Down the Pain

We discussed how SoftWave increases blood flow to an area. And if you have ever looked at a book depicting all the muscles in the body, they are always colored red. They are red because there is a lot of blood in muscle tissue. Muscles need and have a lot of blood flow. And when relaxed, your muscles should be soft and squishy (there's those medical terms again). When there are hard spots or knots in these muscles, this can, at times, be due to lack of blood flow. By squeezing the muscle yourself a bit, you are increasing the blood flow to the area temporarily and creating short-term relief.

Now, imagine a device that can increase that blood flow for you, but at many times greater volume, and deeper than what you can create with your hand or than what you want me to do with my thumb, knuckle, or elbow.

That is what SoftWave does. When I place the applicator on any muscle, the shockwaves that are penetrating the skin and tissue below the skin, i.e., fascia, muscles, and more, immediately create a stimulus to increase blood flow. In a joint, that blood flow can nourish the joint with many different types of molecules that help with inflammation. And in muscles, both superficial and deep, the increased blood flow helps them relax and results in pain relief. And of course, if the muscle is injured, and there is inflammation or a trigger point (trigger points typically have inflammation around the point of pain), SoftWave can address that, as well.

Typically, the trigger point therapy that my fingers, thumbs, or elbows apply on a knot is extremely painful. Just ask my patients. And during the first treatment (before I used SoftWave), I was only able to get to the very superficial aspect of the muscle and attempt to address its surface tension. I will often ask the patients "Who put the cement in that muscle?" because of how hard the muscle felt. Sometimes, it would feel like the whole muscle was tight, and other times there would be a golf-ball-sized area of muscle tension that I would attempt to work out with my aforementioned bony thumbs, knuckles, or elbow. And it would take several visits to reduce or sometimes get rid of the trigger point. Despite what some of my patients may argue, hopefully jokingly, I really don't like causing them unnecessary pain. When I use SoftWave on my patients before doing any manual therapy, the muscle softens significantly so the manual therapy I do afterwards is much less uncomfortable. In addition, I can work on much deeper layers of the muscle in the first visit, which previously wouldn't be accomplished until visits two, three, or four. Working on deeper tissue earlier often results in decreasing the number of times a patient needs to see me.

Ralph's Story is the Perfect Example

Ralph, a male in his seventies, came to me with significant neck pain. He could barely hold his head up by the end of the day. Ralph reported that this had gradually gotten worse over the three to four months prior to seeing me. He was still working full time and planned on doing so until he was seventy-five years old. But at the rate he was going, he did not know if he could keep it up for the next month, much less for the next few years. And if he was forced to retire because of pain, he certainly did not want to spend his retirement feeling like this.

Ralph had to sleep with two or three pillows because his neck hurt so much when he attempted to lie down. What prompted him to see me and trial SoftWave was that the pain had progressed to waking him up each night. He knew he couldn't keep going on as he was, and he did not want to take medications or increase medications that he was already taking.

On inspection of Ralph's posture and neck biomechanics during his first visit with me, I noted that his head sloped forward almost in front of his chest. His shoulders were rounded and also forward. Both of these positions lead to extensive tension in the muscles in his neck and shoulders.

When I palpated his neck muscles, the trapezius muscles literally felt as hard as a rock. His neck and shoulder muscles were extremely tight. On both sides of his neck, I felt major trigger points. As my fingers rolled along the muscles, one side felt like a golf ball and the other was as hard as a golf ball but the size of a quarter. When I pressed on these knots, I could hear him audibly wince. I knew if I dug into these areas, I would be causing him a lot of pain, so I turned to SoftWave.

After applying SoftWave along his upper trapezius and another muscle called the levator scapulae, and inspecting the traps again, there were areas that Ralph reported as tender but not intolerable. As I held the SoftWave applicator over these areas and pressed the dome down on the knots referred to as 'hot spots,' I could feel the areas of the muscle begin to soften. And the beauty of this treatment is that Ralph reported the sensation he was feeling as a "good hurt." When I asked him if it was superficial (close to the surface) or deep, he responded with, "Deep, very deep."

Gradually, as the "good hurt" subsided, an interesting thing happened. Without doing anything else, when I moved to the front of Ralph so I could see how his head was able to move now, Ralph started to sit up straight. He, like many of my patients, looked at me with disbelief.

"What just happened?" he asked.

"SoftWave happened, Ralph," I responded with a smile.

I went on to explain the mechanism of how the increased blood flow that SoftWave caused improved the muscles' ability to work. This blood flow nourished the overworked, overused muscles, and helped them relax and release some tension.

Following the treatment, I was able to further release the trigger points in Ralph's neck without causing him significant pain. We reviewed exercises that he could do at work and at home. When Ralph came in for his next visit, he had a big smile on his face. He said, "I knew that it was working even after the first visit because when I got in my car, I had to adjust the rearview mirror since I was sitting up so much straighter than before."

Over the next three visits, I worked on the mobility of Ralph's neck and shoulders following each SoftWave treatment to improve his biomechanics and posture. By the end of the fourth visit, Ralph was able to sleep through the night and required only one pillow to lay on instead of two or three. He reminds me each time he sees me how grateful he is that he can get a good night's sleep.

But Does SoftWave Work with Chronic Pain?

The last few examples I have given were results of treating patients with SoftWave after:
1. A new injury
2. Pain after a couple of surgeries
3. Pain that was going on for a few months

But how does SoftWave do with pain that has been around for a much longer time, i.e., truly chronic issues?

I'm pretty sure you can guess what I am going to tell you but let me take you through an example anyway.

Meet Molly Fay. She is the talk-show host and Emmy-award-winning broadcast journalist that I referred to before in the example with Susan and her Morton's neuroma. When I started my clinic and brought SoftWave to my area, I had to figure out how to get the word out. Just telling people it worked wasn't going to cut it. It often sounds too good to be true. I had to show people.

I knew that once they came into our office and had a treatment, then the vast majority of people would see the benefit. And if they weren't progressing as they should have by the third visit, then we examined the reasons why. Each of these are explained in this book.

When my first attempts at Facebook and Google ads for my business were a huge failure, I looked for other means of getting the word out. The opportunity to showcase my patients' results, with their permission of course, on a local new show called *The Morning Blend* came to my attention. And honestly, the thought of being on television scared the bajeebies out of me. I had been on TV before, but I found myself wondering, was SoftWave and my patients' experience going to transfer to an interesting segment that could educate patients on the benefits of SoftWave enough that they wanted to come in? And my next question was, would my patients be willing to appear with me on the show?

To my pleasant surprise, the answer was yes on both counts. My patients were eager to tell their stories since they felt better and had more relief than they ever had before, and the producers and hosts at TMJ4 (the station that airs the show) agreed that the topic could be an engaging segment.

Therefore, I began to work with the truly talented people at *The Morning Blend* on TMJ4 every six to eight weeks. These segments were how I survived my first year in business and continue to grow it today. The team at *The Morning Blend* is comprised of individuals who are professional, supportive, and easy to collaborate with. Both of the show hosts, Tiffany Ogle and Molly Fay, are not only experienced and professional, but they are caring journalists who want their guests to succeed. And to my relief, both helped me survive live on-air machine malfunctions, and eased both my stress and the patient's during every show. To check out our shows on *The Morning Blend*, go to this link. https://newyouhealthandwellness.com/morningblendepisodes/.

Over time, after several appearances, an interesting thing started to happen. Molly Fay began to interview me more often than Tiffany. And she started asking me and the guest patient a little bit more about how the treatment worked. She wanted to know how it actually felt. She wanted to know how many treatments they actually needed, and what their longer-term experiences were. Back then, I thought she was helping the segment be more informative, and that is definitely true, but what I did not know was that Molly had an issue with chronic pain herself. And before I knew it, Molly had given our office a call to schedule a trial. After nearly a year of her seeing segment after segment, I was very excited to have her come to the clinic and experience SoftWave herself.

When Molly came to my office on Bluemound Road with an injury that had been plaguing her for over ten years, I'm not going to lie: I was a little nervous. SoftWave is phenomenal when it comes to acute or chronic joint and muscle pain, but when symptoms like Molly's have been around for over a decade, I just never know. I am always very honest with my patients. My brain always wonders what else could be going on when a seemingly healthy person is still experiencing pain and swelling in an area that should have healed years ago.

I could go on and explain Molly's experience from my perspective, but she's the journalist, so I'll let her take it from here.

From Molly Fay

After interviewing Stacey multiple times on **The Morning Blend,** I decided it was time to see if this SoftWave thing could help me. She introduced us to so many patients who had success stories. Stacey helped them with all sorts of problems, from pelvic floor issues and chronic shoulder pain to plantar fasciitis and ED. My left ankle had been bothering me for years. Could she get the swelling down and make it hurt less? If I'm being honest, I was doubtful. I did not doubt her experience and expertise. I doubted the treatment itself because I had tried everything: physical therapy, ultrasound treatments, massage, dry needling, and anti-inflammatory drugs. Years ago, I also had an MRI and considered surgery every time the swelling became severe or the pain became intense.

At my first visit, I was impressed and a bit shocked by how much time Stacey spent with me. This was no ordinary doctor or PT visit. She wanted to know more than just when I first hurt my ankle and what treatments I had already tried. She was interested in things like nutrition, recent bloodwork results, the types of activities that aggravated my ankle problem, and even what shoes I wore every day. In fact, she asked me to bring in my shoes so she could see them! Now I understand. Footwear is an important part of maintaining the gains her patients make with treatment. Shouldn't all health professionals care more about that kind of stuff? That's probably a topic for another book!

Back to my ankle. Stacey has already explained SoftWave therapy and how it works in detail. I can't add much to that, but I can tell you my initial impression was that it wouldn't work. The machine looked ordinary. If it wasn't about an injection, cutting my ankle open, or making it hurt, how could it work? Then Stacey said something I've never heard anyone else say on my ankle journey. She said that if it was going to work, I would probably know that day–in her office–after the first treatment. She did not guarantee that it would be perfectly good as new, but she said I should notice some type of improvement. On day one. My thoughts were that it was a bold statement, perhaps too optimistic, but I was open to it because I wanted to heal.

The treatment is not painful, but it's a little uncomfortable in certain spots. It feels like a gentle tap in some areas and then a little more like a hammer in su-per sensitive areas. I'm not sure how else to explain it, but during the whole treatment, Stacey checks in to make sure it's tolerable. It's definitely tolerable! My guess is that those sensitive spots are exactly where inflammation is most pronounced. That's where SoftWave needs to be! Stacey explained the science behind it. So, I will just add this: the swelling went down NOTICEABLY after that first ten-minute SoftWave treatment and Stacey's manual therapy! The swelling remained that way until my next visit, too. I agreed to wear good shoes with good support. That helped. In addition to the SoftWave, Stacey also suggested we try a compression boot.

Those two treatments in combination started producing really good results. My swelling continued to improve with several more sessions and the pain was so much less. In fact, I was able to walk five miles in Charleston, South Carolina, on an anniversary trip with my husband–pain free! I got new Vionic sneakers before that trip and I'm sure that helped, but those treatments gave me back an activity I love. I have always loved walking, but I wasn't doing it anymore, except to walk the dog and things like that. Even now, months later, the swelling is still so much less. At one time it looked like the foot of an elephant, now it looks almost exactly like my other ankle. Nothing else I have ever tried for my ankle has worked as well as SoftWave. I also had a similar experience when Stacey used SoftWave and her program to treat my plantar fasciitis. It was debilitating at times and to my delight, with Stacey's help, I was able to eliminate that, too.

My story would not be complete without also telling you about my shoulder. For a few years, I struggled with shoulder pain on the right side. I had considered PT, but always assumed it was related to something peri-menopausal because so many women report feeling joint pain and muscle stiffness. Then on December 20, 2022, I fell. My right shoulder hurt so much that I cried most of the night, visited urgent care the next day, and took a week off work. I couldn't raise my arm more than chest high and I was in constant pain. I did PT for several months and got some of my mobility back, but the pain continued. My doctor recommended an MRI, and it turns out I had a massive, full-thickness tear in my rotator cuff. Two tendons were completely severed and retracted. So, on February 20, 2023, I had rotator cuff surgery.

Anyone who has had rotator cuff surgery can tell you that the recovery is both painful and long. About six weeks after surgery, I returned to PT. I made progress and was able to return to walking and light household chores. Eventually, I was able to ditch the sling, too. After about twelve weeks, I also returned to work. Stacey checked in with me regularly, asking about my progress. She also mentioned that I could try SoftWave if my PT and surgeon agreed it was okay. Stacey said it might be particularly useful if my progress stalled.

Once again, Stacey was right. I hit a plateau and was really struggling with rotating my arm at the shoulder. It had been several weeks since I had made any progress in regular PT. To my surprise, both my physical therapist and my surgeon gave me the thumbs up to try SoftWave. It was so reassuring that all of the people involved in my care agreed on this! After my first SoftWave visit with Stacey, guess what?! I got some of my mobility back and the progress continued.

I was pleasantly surprised that SoftWave was not painful, either. My other PT agreed that this progress was noticeable and probably due to SoftWave. It's important for me to note that Stacey used more than SoftWave at these visits. She incorporated manual therapy in my treatments. I'd like to say that it was not intense, but I'd be lying. The best way I can describe manual therapy is significant stretching of what Stacey called 'the capsule' of the shoulder. In my case, after surgery, the capsule of my shoulder was getting tight. Stacey said the capsule is like a balloon that surrounds the shoulder and keeps the fluid that nourishes the shoulder inside it.

Because I hadn't been able to move my shoulder through its full range for a while, the capsule shrunk and made it harder to get the motion back. The manual therapy she did was meant to stretch the capsule. Stacey used SoftWave to bring blood flow to that capsule so that it was easier to stretch. It involved stretching the shoulder joint in all different positions with Stacey applying pressure on certain muscles to encourage normal movement. My other physical therapist said I had plateaued significantly at least twice. Both times I returned to SoftWave therapy, and it turned things around and got my shoulder moving again, increasing my range of motion. I was truly afraid I wouldn't be able to move my shoulder normally again without pain, but now my shoulder is almost normal, and I am back to doing yoga and strength training.

SoftWave and the program Stacey put together for me has honestly been a game changer for my ankle and my shoulder. I am forever thankful to have had this treatment.

I am happy to report that Molly's experience is not an exception but often the rule, especially when the pain and inflammation is localized/tangible due to triggers that can be addressed with SoftWave and a comprehensive rehabilitation strategy, not just a handout with exercises on it.

You are Going to Put That Where? SoftWave and Pelvic Pain

Janice sat across from me, and I have to admit there were times in my evaluation of her situation that I had to fight back tears.

Referred to me from a friend who knew I had a SoftWave machine and recommended to me because I am a pelvic health therapist, Janice was a woman in her late thirties with two children. She described the strain on her marriage and the guilt she felt at times when she started to experience vaginismus, a disorder that results in such fear of having intercourse due to pain that it becomes physically impossible.

"I am afraid I am losing my husband," she said, as she reached for a tissue in the box on my desk.

I swallowed hard and felt my eyes blinking excessively as she went on to explain the difficulty she had after a medical procedure to attempt to improve incontinence after her last child was born.

"It felt like glass shards were ripping through my vagina whenever we tried to attempt having sex. Eventually, we just stopped trying. We both thought it was a temporary thing and I just needed more time to heal after the procedure, but years went by and still nothing has changed."

When I asked Janice if she ever had pelvic floor physical therapy before, she said she had and with good results. But within three months of finishing the therapy, despite following through with all that she had been taught, the pain slowly came back, and she was in the same situation again.

After mentioning the pelvic floor specialist she saw, I knew she had seen a very experienced practitioner for whom I have a lot of respect. Therefore, the quality of the therapy wasn't the problem.

I told Janice about SoftWave, and that I had been the first physical therapist in the country to consistently utilize it for pelvic floor disorders for both men and women, and that I had been running a study on dyspareunia (painful intercourse) that was approved by an Institutional Review Board (IRB). Unfortunately, due to exclusion criteria involved with the study, Janice did not qualify, but that did not exclude her from SoftWave treatment outside of the research study.

What Is an Institutional Review Board (IRB)?

An IRB is also called an independent ethics committee, an ethical review board, or a research ethics board. It is an administrative body established to protect the rights and welfare of human research subjects recruited to participate in research activities conducted under the institution to which it is affiliated.

We talked about how the pelvic floor can be a significant problem when patients have pain with intercourse, and she said she would be okay with an internal assessment.

I stepped out of the room to let Janice got herself ready for the treatment.

A few minutes went by, and I knocked on the door, cracked it slightly, and asked, "All set?"

"Yep," she answered, and I walked in.

As Janice lay comfortably under the grey sheets, I rolled my stool up to the side of the treatment table, and we talked about the internal assessment, and that she was able to stop at any time if it was too painful.

I instructed her in diaphragmatic breathing exercises that she could do to settle her nervous system. She was already familiar with them from her last PT. She started breathing deeply, and immediately I saw her belly rise with inhaling and fall with exhaling, so I knew she was a pro.

While the internal assessment was not thorough due to her intense pain, I was able to palpate significant tone in the muscles of the pelvic floor, and I also noticed tension when I checked a few muscles externally. Even external palpation induced significant discomfort.

Next, I explained how SoftWave worked, and that the treatment was completely external. Unlike any other modality or shockwave device, the waves from SoftWave could penetrate deep and wide enough to get to all three layers of the pelvic floor without provoking her pain. She agreed to have the treatment done.

I took her through step by step how SoftWave brings blood flow immediately to the tissue that was 'upregulated,' resulting in muscle tone or tension release.

Next, I showed her the applicator and her eyes got a bit big, and she asked, "You are going to put that where?"

I gently rested my hand on her forearm and reminded her this was a completely external treatment. I went on to let her know she may not feel anything but a gentle tapping and a wave into her pelvic floor. If she did have any discomfort from the wave, we would adjust the intensity to her tolerance and could stop at ANY time during the treatment.

"Are you ready?" I asked.

"Ready as I'll ever be," she responded.

We placed the applicator first on her hand so she could feel the tapping.

"Oh, that's not bad," said Janice.

I also showed her what if felt like on a fleshier area on her stomach.

"All good?" I asked.

"Yeah, I think so," she said.

Then with her knee bent and relaxed out to the side, I placed the applicator, covered with a transparent cap and ultrasound gel, on her perineum, the area between the anus and the vagina.

We started at a low level of intensity, and when she felt ready, we increased the energy until she felt the wave penetrating.

"How are you doing?" I asked above the clicking noise.

"Pretty good," she replied, with a puzzled look on her face. "I've never felt anything like this before."

"That's what all of my patients say." After a short pause, I asked, "Are you having any pain?"

"No, not pain. And that surprises me. It's like," she paused. "I feel the wave you were talking about and the tapping. When you point it that way," she pointed to her left, "I can feel it up to my hip bone. It's not pain, but I can definitely feel it." She paused again and looked at me. "Shouldn't I feel pain?"

"Not necessarily." I explained, "The pelvic floor consists of three layers of muscles, and when you have pain with intercourse like you do, those muscles can go into protective mode, holding a certain amount of tension or tone continuously."

Janice nodded. "I do remember my other PT saying something like that."

"And when that happens over a long period of time, those muscles aren't getting the blood flow they need to relax fully. So SoftWave, because it penetrates wide and deep, almost immediately starts bringing more blood to the whole area, and those muscles can finally let go."

After about ten minutes, we finished the treatment, and I asked if I could try an internal assessment again.

"You can try," Janice answered, giving me the go-ahead after shrugging her shoulders

As I began the internal exam, I asked, "Are you okay?"

Her eyes immediately became glassy. "That," she replied, with a blank expression on her face, "that doesn't hurt." A single tear fell from the corner of each of her eyes.

I was able to perform some internal work on the pelvic floor to attempt reduce the tone or tension further.

There was only one spot where she mentioned the sensation felt like a slight burning but was not uncomfortable. After I completed the treatment, we sat in silence for a few moments as she wept.

"I'm sorry," she said, as she took a deep breath in. "It's just that it's been so long since I haven't had any pain, you know . . . there."

"Absolutely no apology necessary," I responded.

Janice continued with three more treatments and was happy to report that she was able to have intercourse again with her husband. This is significant, as many times, treatments for vaginismus can easily take ten or more sessions to find some relief. During her last session with me, Janice mentioned that she and her husband decided to go to couple's therapy, as they realized there was more than just a lack of intercourse that was causing problems in their relationship. I let her know I was so happy for them.

I kept in touch with Janice for a few months to make sure she was still doing well. The last time I reached out, I was taken by surprise when I heard a male voice on the other end of the call. "Hello, Stacey?" the gruff voice asked.

Ah, yes, this is Stacey. I was looking for Janice." I checked my phone screen to see if I dialed the wrong number.

"Hey, yes, Janice is here. This is Dean, her husband."

"Oh, hi, Dean. It's nice to *sort of* meet you."

"I saw your name pop up on Janice's phone. She is just downstairs."

"Okay, please have her call me back. It was nice to . . ."

Dean interrupted me, "Hey, I picked up because I wanted to say something to you."

"Okay," I replied, as my stomach tightened slightly.

"I just wanted to say, uh, thanks."

A short silence fell between us, and I took a deep breath and slowly let it out.

"I just wanted to say," Dean repeated as he cleared his throat. "Yeah, thanks for giving me my wife back."

It's moments like this that make me so incredibly grateful for being able to do what I do, and equally grateful that Laura, my friend of forty-plus years, reminded me to be open-minded and focus on the possibilities instead of being cynical and making decisions only on past experiences. SoftWave has truly changed my life and has improved the lives of many of my patients. I continue to help SoftWave create new protocols and expand on research, so more people looking for answers, like Janice and her husband Dean, may someday reap the benefits of this incredible technology.

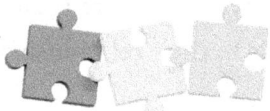

Key Pieces

Different Shockwave Devices/Different Outcomes: Not all shockwave devices are created equal, or even produce a shockwave, so the buyer and patient must beware. Typically, if a practitioner says there is no difference between shockwave devices, they don't understand the technology. A practitioner should know the indications and limitations of their devices based on current research and they should accurately convey that to the patient.

SoftWave Therapy Benefits: SoftWave therapy has shown promise in treating a variety of pain conditions, from acute injuries to chronic issues, often providing relief where other treatments have failed.

Technology Evolution: The distinction between true shockwave devices and radial pressure wave devices is crucial for patient comfort and outcomes.

Impact on Patients' Lives: SoftWave therapy has significantly improved the quality of life for many patients, offering a completely noninvasive, comfortable treatment for relief from chronic pain and enabling people to resume activities they love.

Want to see if SoftWave Can Help You?
In the Southeastern Wisconsin area, call 414-299-8121or email info@newyouhealthandwellness.com

Outside of Southeastern Wisconsin? Go to https://softwavetrt.com/providers/ to search for a provider in your area.

CHAPTER 8

Tackling the Intangible Triggers

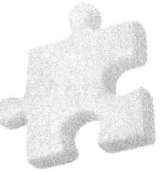

"Hope sees the invisible, feels the intangible, and achieves the impossible."

—Helen Keller

As Jim sat across from me after seeing an ad for our services on Facebook, I could hear the faint tapping of my fingers as they roared across my keyboard while Jim discussed his past medical history, the supplements he was taking, his current complaints, and how he hurt his hip. His face cringed a bit as he contorted his body, trying to recreate what had happened when he fell on his deck two summers ago.

"I landed right on it," he explained. "And it did not hurt much after I got up. But when I woke up the next morning, it hurt like hell."

"Does it hurt right now, sitting here?" I asked.

He wiggled around in his seat. "I mean, not really," he replied, his eyes looking up and away as he leaned over on the side of his injury. "Well, maybe a little bit." He met my eyes again. "It really only hurts a lot if I bend over."

Before I knew it, Jim was up out of his seat and attempting to touch his toes. "Yeah, right there."

His right hand was patting his right hip as he rose up slowly.

"What number would you give that pain?" So many of my patients hate that question.

"I don't know." He bent over again and slowly came back up to standing. "A five or a six?"

"Okay," I said, as I watched Jim take his seat again on the black upholstered chair in front of my desk. "Has it been a five to six out of ten since you injured it?"

"No, not really. It went away a few weeks after I hurt it. But then, these past few months, it has come back." He paused, then continued, "It started to hurt at night and woke me up a couple of times; then I noticed it when I started up my workouts again."

After that, our conversation, which was geared toward gathering as much information as I could about Jim's issue, ended and we moved toward my evaluation of how his body moved. I palpated his sacroiliac joint when he bent over again, and I looked at whether his hips stayed level when he stood on one leg. I asked him to walk around as I observed his gait pattern.

We moved to the table, and it was time to assess his flexibility. Jim winced a little when I slowly picked his straight leg up in the air. His leg felt heavy, and I found myself lifting against quite a bit of resistance.

"My hamstrings have always been so tight."

"Ah, yeah, I can see that," I replied, as I smiled and moved my feet a little farther apart to stabilize myself to see how far his long leg would allow me to lift it.

I found the same tightness in the other leg, as well. The muscles that rotate both hips were tight, too. But these weren't issues that just happened with his injury a couple of summers ago, and the long-standing tightness in his muscles now could be exacerbating his current hip pain.

I palpated right over his hip bone on the side of his leg, and his face crinkled up. "Yep, that's another spot."

I was right over the bursa of the hip. A bursa is a common structure found around joints. They can act as shock absorbers and provide a little extra padding and protection to the bony parts of our body and help tendons slide over and around bones with ease. With pain directly on this area, his diagnosis of 'bursitis' from his primary care doctor was confirmed. But the pieces of the puzzle that did not fit were why the pain would have come back without any recurrence of an injury, and why was it waking him up occasionally at night?

X-rays had ruled out any issue with the bone itself, and an MRI also ruled out any serious pathology. That test simply showed some inflammation in the area where Jim had his pain, but not enough for the doctor to be overly concerned.

Part of me thought the hip pain would resolve with our advanced technology called SoftWave, the modality that you learned about in Chapter 7. This, coupled with soft tissue work on his muscles, much-needed flexibility exercises for his hips and back, stabilization exercises for his core and hip, and possibly some support in his shoes were probably what would help Jim knock out the niggling pain in his back and hip. So, we started Jim's weekly program.

But the other part of me knew, after looking at his information that included digestive problems, fatigue, and issues with sleeping that had developed long before his current back pain that there may be other areas that we would need to investigate if this pain did not go away. I mentioned this to Jim in his first appointment, and he seemed a bit dismissive of there being any other reason for his pain besides the previous injury. He was excited to get started with the program to treat his hip and back directly and work toward getting rid of his pain.

Jim was delighted to find some relief after his first treatment. As a matter of fact, right after our first session together, he was able to bend over without pain. When I saw Jim again the following week, he reported that he slept like a baby the night after the treatment, but the pain slowly came back after two days. This is a typical response after one full treatment session, so we were both happy that he responded well.

After his second visit, Jim was glad to report the pain was gone again. He promised that he was religious with his exercises, and I could see some changes in his strength and flexibility, so I knew he wasn't simply giving me lip service.

He reported that the aching came back one night, and sometimes randomly during the day, but overall, it was at least 50 percent better and he was happy with the progress ... that is, until I saw him the next week.

When Jim came back for visit number three, he seemed despondent. His brow was heavy and furrowed when he arrived in the treatment room.

"Hey Jim, what's going on? How are you?" I asked, expecting to hear good news.

"It's back," he replied, as he sunk into the office chair with a thump.

"It's back?" I asked.

"Yes!" He threw his hands up in the air. "I don't understand it. Everything was going so well, but it's right back to where it was when I first came in."

"What number out of ten would you say it is now?" I asked.

"I don't really feel it right now." True to form, Jim jumped up to test it out and bent over. "Last night while I was working out, it was back to at least a four." His chest heaved with frustration.

"Okay, looking back when you first came in, when you bent over, the pain was about a five to six out of ten. And now it's a four?"

"Yeah, but for those two weeks after we started the treatment, it was like a two, and sometimes even a zero. And it's back to waking me up at night. I don't know." He avoided eye contact. "Maybe this just isn't working."

I asked him what had gone on over the last week since I had seen him. He couldn't think of anything different that he had done, and he promised he hadn't overdone it at his workouts.

I believed him.

My next question was, did he change his sleep pattern, increase alcohol consumption, eat any differently, get new shoes? Was anything different?

"What would any of that have to do with my hip and back pain?" he asked.

"Well," I went on to explain, "remember what we talked about at the first visit. I asked you all those questions about your digestion, your energy levels, your bowel function, etc."

"Yes, I remember. I thought it was weird that you would ask about that stuff when I came to see you for my hip."

"Do you remember that I mentioned there could be other causes contributing to the inflammation in the joint, and how your hip and back really should have been healed by now since the injury was a couple of years ago?"

"I guess."

"Well, I think there might be some other contributing factors to the pain you are experiencing. Other causes of the inflammation."

He stared at me without saying a word.

"Okay, let's go over that again. If what we are doing in the clinic helps when you are here and lasts for a few hours to a few days, that is a good sign that what we are doing is helping your body move through the inflammatory process, and hopefully either decreasing the inflammation enough that you don't feel it or even helping the body heal on its own. Remember the example of the scratch on your hand?"

"Yeah, yeah, if I keep scratching it, it won't get better. I remember."

"With the first two treatments, we were making progress and eliminating the triggers that we thought were causing inflammation in the area that you had pain. True?"

"True."

"We had also been working on the tangible triggers away from the area of pain. Your flexibility in the hip, knee, calf, and back. As well as muscle strength in some of those areas."

"Yep."

"We talked about the biomechanics (how your body was moving) and corrected some movements to further remove the stress from the painful area, including looking at your shoes and making sure they gave you a good foundation to support the lower extremities, pelvis, hip, and back. And we've ruled out any serious bulging disc from the MRI, and even exercises that would help or hurt you if it was a disc issue."

"Yes, I understand, we did all that, but why did the pain come back after we were doing so well?"

"It did not come back to quite the same intensity as before, but the fact that it came back must be extremely frustrating. I get it. But I do see this about 20 to 30 percent of the time when an injury from a year or more ago slowly and for no apparent reason comes back or comes and goes without steady progress. I also see this with very old injuries that are not making progress at all. When we see this recurrence of pain without a reinjury, we have to start asking ourselves what else can be triggering inflammation that is causing the pain to recur."

"I thought you said that is what we are doing."

"Yes, we are. But what if inflammation in the joint was a result of something other than just how you are moving? What if there's another trigger or triggers?"

"You mean like arthritis?"

"No, not exactly. Arthritis or inflammation in the joint due to joint damage could definitely be a part of the problem, but if it was just arthritis, why would it hurt sometimes and not others? Or why would it disturb your sleep some nights and not others, if you haven't been any more active one day than another day?"

Jim stared at me. And I thought I might be losing him.

"Think of it this way. Imagine a pitcher filling up with water from a couple of faucets running into it. The water represents the inflammation in your hip. When you are here, with our treatment, we pour out the water (inflammation) and turn off the faucets (triggers) that we think are the culprits. Then the inflammation should go away because the body is finally able to heal."

"Okay, I see that."

"But what if there's another source of inflammation? What if there's another faucet that we couldn't see or that we did not notice that is slowly filling up the pitcher?"

The skin tensed on his forehead.

I continued. "What if there was another culprit; one or even more we haven't addressed? And it's causing water to fill up the pitcher slowly over time after we empty it, like a slow drip in the plumbing at your house that is hard to find. You can't pin down where it's coming from. If you empty the pitcher and don't find all the sources that are filling it up, in our case the other trigger or triggers, then even if you pour the pitcher out every night, it would eventually fill up again."

"Okay, that part makes sense, but how do we find that?"

"Trying to figure out if there is another source of inflammation in the body that is causing inflammation in a joint is not as easy as seeing and addressing the obvious triggers like your muscle weakness and tightness, or adjusting how you are moving. For example, if the inflammation is systemic, it can be coming from one of several different sources other than the joint where you have the pain."

Jim threw his hands up in the air, and they landed hard on the arms of the chair. "Well, just tell me what the heck you think it is and let's do something about it. I can't go on living like this. If this isn't going to work, I might as well go back and get another cortisone injection."

"Yes, you could do that. But remember what we talked about. Cortisone has now been shown to be related to increasing degeneration in your joints, potentially because it is stopping or significantly slowing down your body's own healing process."

"Yeah, but at least it might give me some relief."

"You are right. It might. But it isn't addressing the reason why the pain keeps coming back, though, is it?"

"No. I guess it isn't."

"Here's the deal. Of the people I see who do everything from a biomechanical point of view to take the obvious triggers away from irritating the joint, this fixes joint and muscle pain for approximately 70 to 80 percent of the patients. But when my patients experience what you have been describing to me:

- Aching at night without a reinjury or significantly increased activity
- Pain relieved for a short period or even a long period of time and then coming back for seemingly no reason
- Pain that is not relieved even though they are doing everything that they are supposed to be doing
- There's no apparent reason for the pain or symptoms based on X-rays, MRIs, or other scans

"When I see your scenario, i.e., despite addressing your biomechanics, and using shockwave, and doing soft tissue work, your pain isn't continuing to improve, and you have other symptoms such as:

- Fatigue
- Digestive issues (constipation, diarrhea, bloating)
- Mood changes
- Other pain in the muscles and joints not resolving
- Difficulty losing weight despite trying everything
- Cravings at night
- Sleep issues

We need to start thinking outside the box."

"Okay, like what?"

"I suggest we start considering other factors that new research has shown can be linked to chronic and acute muscle and joint pain. These factors are:

- The gut-joint axis
- How foods can impact joint health
- Hormones and how they impact pain sensitivity and joint health
- Pain science: how the brain impacts and perpetuates chronic pain"

"I don't really understand any of that or how it has anything to do with my back and hip pain. But I am at my wits' end. You were my last resort. I've tried everything, and even though the pain isn't gone completely so far, we at least have seen some positive changes unlike anything else I have done in the past. So, if you think there is something else we should look at, then just tell me what blood tests to get, and I'll have my doctor order them."

"I wish it were that easy. There are blood tests to measure inflammation in the body, but they are not specific to the joints. And there are a few blood tests that can measure levels of antibodies in the blood that indicate certain autoimmune diseases that may affect the joints, but you don't have the symptoms to make me think you have rheumatoid arthritis, lupus, or other autoimmune issues. Finally, there is one test to measure uric acid in the body, but this is related to a disease called gout."

"I don't have gout," Jim replied.

"Yes, I know, that was just an example of blood tests that are available but not related to your situation."

Common Tests That Measure Inflammation in the Body

- C-Reactive Protein (CRP): CRP is a protein produced by the liver in response to inflammation. High levels of CRP in the blood can indicate acute or chronic inflammation, suggesting an underlying condition such as infections, autoimmune diseases, or chronic diseases. There are two types of CRP tests: a standard CRP test, which can detect wide-range inflammation, and a high-sensitivity CRP (hs-CRP) test, which is used to assess the risk of cardiovascular disease.
- Erythrocyte Sedimentation Rate (ESR): The ESR test measures the rate at which red blood cells sediment in a period of one hour. A faster-than-normal rate may indicate inflammation in the body. ESR is not specific to any one disease but can be elevated in the presence of inflammation, infection, autoimmune diseases, and chronic conditions.
- Complete Blood Count (CBC): While not specifically an inflammation test, the CBC can provide indirect signs of inflammation. For example, an increased white blood cell count (leukocytosis) can indicate infection or inflammation, and other components of the CBC can provide additional clues about the underlying cause.
- Ferritin: Ferritin is a protein that stores iron in the body. Levels can become elevated in the presence of inflammation, as the body may increase ferritin production in response to stress or injury. Elevated ferritin levels can be seen in conditions such as rheumatoid arthritis, hemochromatosis, and liver disease.

Tests specifically for joint inflammation and autoimmune issues:

- Rheumatoid Factor (RF): RF is an antibody found in the blood of many people with rheumatoid arthritis (RA) and some other autoimmune diseases. While not specific to RA, a high level of RF can suggest this condition.
- Antinuclear Antibodies (ANA): The presence of ANAs can indicate an autoimmune disorder, such as lupus (systemic lupus erythematosus (SLE)) or Sjögren's syndrome. ANAs are not specific to any one autoimmune disease but can signal the immune system's abnormal activity against the body's own cells.

> - Uric Acid: Elevated levels of uric acid can suggest gout, a type of inflammatory arthritis that results from the crystallization of uric acid within the joints, leading to intense pain and swelling.

"So, unless there was a disease process like an autoimmune issue or gout, both of which are always accompanied by systemic inflammation and usually have blood tests to help confirm the diagnosis, there isn't a reliable test to help determine exactly where joint pain like yours is coming from if those diagnoses have been ruled out."

"Alright, for heaven's sake, what is the next step?"

Intangible Triggers

"The next step is to identify the intangible triggers of inflammation and address these," I replied.

"Intangible what?" he asked.

"Intangible triggers. These are the triggers of inflammation that are not easily measured, but when addressed and mostly or completely eliminated, your joint, muscle, or in your case likely bursitis (inflammation of the bursa) can go away for good."

Jim stared at me, with his brow crinkled and his head cocked to one side.

"Jim, would you agree that this pain is affecting your emotions and moods? It's affecting the way you function socially. You have said that you aren't going out with friends like you used to or reaching out to family like before you were injured. Isn't that true?"

His eyes welled up and he moved his gaze away from mine. "Maybe." He took a deep breath in through his nose and exhaled. "Yeah, yeah, it is." He looked back at me.

Jim finally started to come around to the idea that there was something else going on than just the pain in one localized area. After all, he had tried everything, and though SoftWave and our program was the first intervention that gave him some relief, the relief was not long-lasting. My hope was that our conversation would help him realize that the pain was now starting to affect his life in many ways. This was not solely a biological problem anymore. It was affecting all aspects of his life, including his social connections and his mental health. This is not uncommon with chronic pain, and conventional medicine has talked about this for more than fifty years. It's called the Bio-psycho-social model related to pain. Thankfully, I am starting to see conventional medicine practitioners talking with their patients more about this.

What Is the Bio-Psycho-Social Model?

Bio-psycho-social means pain can be complex and not simply be a result of an injury or a problem that can be identified on an X-ray or MRI. You've learned in previous chapters that often times, especially for low back pain or pelvic pain, what's identified on MRI is not what is causing the pain. In recent years, most doctors are coming around to accepting the fact that pain is multidimensional.

There can be a biological source (tangible from an injury or biomechanical issue or intangible trigger, i.e., systemic inflammation)

There can be a psychological source, especially when the pain is associated with significant emotional distress.

There can be a social source, meaning there is significant functional disability that impacts a person's daily life, hobbies, and participation in social events or roles.

The next step after addressing the physical, tangible triggers is to assess the intangible triggers:

1. The gut-joint axis and food sensitivities
2. Hormone levels
3. Stress
4. The brain and pain connection

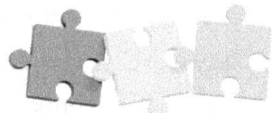

Key Pieces

Beyond Tangible Triggers: Chronic pain may persist even after addressing tangible triggers. Identifying intangible triggers from the assessment of gut health (gut-joint axis and gut-muscle axis), eating plan/food sensitivities, hormone levels, emotional stress, and chronic pain's impact on the brain are areas that have a significant influence on finally relieving chronic pain.

Chronic Pain is Often Multidimensional: It involves biological, psychological, and social factors, all of which must be considered in treatment.

Comprehensive Approach Needed: When traditional treatments aren't enough, exploring a holistic approach that looks outside of the conventional system often creates a roadmap to relief.

CHAPTER 9
Gut Health and Joint/Muscle Pain

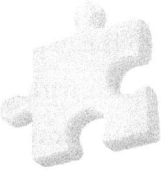

"The gut is not like Las Vegas—what happens in the gut does not stay in the gut."

–Dr. Alessio Fasano

After meeting the libero's forearms, the white leather ball reversed course as it soared gracefully into the air. It paused momentarily at the peak of its arc, as if suspended by invisible threads, before falling toward the fingertips of the player standing on the wooden gym floor whose right shoulder sat perpendicular to the volleyball net. There, the setter set the ball with deft precision, aligning it perfectly for the five-foot-eleven blonde hitter who slammed it down across the net for a decisive kill. Jean's heart surged as she sprung to her feet with pride. Her daughter sprinted back to her teammates; her hands triumphantly thrown up in the air.

The vibrant cheers echoing from the court sliced through Jean like a double-edged sword. They were a stark reminder of a time when her own movements mirrored the athletes before her—swift, seamless, and unburdened by pain. Now, as Jean attempted to return to the wooden bleacher below her, she braced herself for the familiar pain in her knee as she lowered herself. It was hard to discern whether the creaks she was hearing were from the bleachers as the rest of the fans returned to their seats, or from her swollen and sore knee. Jean let out a deep breath as her bottom rested on the hard seat.

Since the set was almost over, her gaze drifted to the stairs at an arm's length beside her. She dreaded shuffling between the long benches and then descending the stairs when the match was over. Her muscles braced at the thought of the familiar pain with every movement: sometimes a sharp, piercing jolt and other times a deep, gnawing ache that seemed to have taken permanent residence in her knee. You met Jean in Chapter 1 of this book, after her doctor had diagnosed her with severe osteoarthritis, telling her that her knee was "bone on bone," and only a total knee replacement would relieve the pain she was experiencing.

The Plateau and a New Direction

Back at home, Jean's living room was scattered with various orthopedic aids, stark evidence of her long battle with knee pain. Despite diligent adherence to physical therapy, regular changes in footwear, and a host of cortisone injections over the years, the relief was fleeting. She could still feel the intense flare-ups that followed her long days on her feet walking from classroom to classroom. It was becoming increasingly clear that surface-level treatments were not enough. That is when she showed up in my office.

Jean's appointment unfolded much like those of many patients who walk through our doors. We began with a thorough discussion about medications, lifestyle, past medical history, and her current circumstances. Yet, Jean's visit was underscored by a particularly pressing concern: her fervent desire to avoid knee replacement surgery. Her resolve was deeply rooted in personal history—her mother's arduous journey through two revision surgeries, following promises of pain relief that never materialized after the initial procedure. This family history sharpened Jean's determination to find an alternative path to healing.

I assessed her biomechanics in an attempt to identify any tangible triggers contributing to ongoing pain. Indeed, she had weak hip stabilizers, tight calf muscles, and an arch that continued to fall when she walked up stairs, despite her custom-fit orthotics from a podiatrist. Upon visual inspection and palpation of her knee, I noticed it was warm and swollen, clearly indicating she was stuck in the proinflammatory stage. Jean reported these symptoms as normal.

Following our first SoftWave treatment, there was a glimmer of hope. Jean stood up from the treatment table and noted much less pain. Her limp was gone, and the swelling had visibly decreased. Her face beamed, and her eyes brightened. "Maybe this will work," she commented.

After the first two visits, Jean returned to the clinic. As she entered the treatment room, I could see the limp was still apparent but looked less severe. She slowly sat down in the chair across from me, and after I asked how she was doing, Jean reported, "The pain is better."

"On a scale of zero to ten, where ten would mean you would want to go to the emergency room, what level of pain are you having at rest?" I asked.

"About a three to four," Jean replied.

"That is a bit better," I replied. "And with stairs?"

She hesitated. Her eyes looked off into the distance as both hands rubbed her knee. Her gaze landed back on me. "That can get up to an eight at times."

My heart sank a bit in my chest. "So, no change with the stairs?"

"Not really," she replied.

I asked if she was doing the taping of both her arch and her kneecap that we started during the last treatment. She nodded. I asked if she was performing her exercises for her hip and stretching for her calves.

"As much as I can," she replied.

"Does it still ache at night as much as it did before? And does it wake you up?"

"That may be slightly better, but yes, it still aches, some nights more than others."

"Would you say that it aches more on days you walk more?"

"No, not really. I do about the same amount of walking every day at school."

"If you don't have significant relief after this treatment, we need to look at other areas. So, between now and your next visit, I would like you to keep a food diary and a symptom diary."

I gestured toward the worksheet I slid toward her. "Please keep track of everything on that sheet. Write down everything you are eating and drinking, your activity levels, and your symptoms."

Jean pulled her reading glasses from the top of her head, reached out her hand, took the paper from the table, and began to inspect it.

She responded with an, "Ah, okay." A few minutes later, she looked up at me over her readers and asked, "What will this tell you about my knee?"

Understanding the Gut-Joint Axis

Imagine your body as a bustling metropolitan area, where the gut is the main post office that communicates with neighborhoods full of inhabitants. The gut-joint axis functions like the capital city's postal system, efficiently sending biochemical messages between the gastrointestinal tract (the post office) and the joints (houses in the neighborhood). The messages travel via the blood and even in the spaces in between cells. This system sends nourishment and other molecules to many areas inside the body.

This sophisticated communication is managed by the gut microbiota, an incredibly diverse community of microbes (bacteria) residing in the gut. Each microbe and group of microbes plays a specific role, akin to citizens in the capital city, contributing to the overall health and functionality of the body.

Besides the joints, the gut also communicates with:

- The brain (gut-brain axis)
- The liver (gut-liver axis)
- The skin (gut-skin axis)
- The lungs (gut-lung axis)
- The kidneys (gut-kidney axis)
- The heart (gut-heart axis)

Research is emerging every day that shows the importance of the relationship of the gut with *all* the organ systems of the body.

Research Supporting the Gut-Joint Connection

Recent research has illuminated the significant role of the gut microbiota in maintaining joint health, and its potential impact on inflammatory diseases like osteoarthritis and rheumatoid arthritis. Several studies now highlight that an imbalance in the gut microbiota, known as dysbiosis, can lead to the development of pro-inflammatory states that are associated with rheumatoid arthritis. This dysbiosis can alter immune responses, increasing systemic inflammation that directly affects joint health.

But many have questioned whether the gut could impact the development of osteoarthritis, often thought of as a localized wear-and-tear issue. Then, one of the first studies to confirm the relationship between the gut and joint health came along. The research revealed a direct correlation with a key proinflammatory product found in the gut. This product was elevated in the joints of people with osteoarthritis. A review of additional evidence shows the gut-joint axis is multifactorial, but these products from the gut, referred to as lipopolysaccharides (LPS), when elevated, are believed to wreak havoc in joints and other areas of the body. Subsequent studies have confirmed this phenomenon, but this may just be the tip of the iceberg.

Lipopolysaccharides (LPS)

Lipopolysaccharides (LPS) are a part of gram-negative bacteria found in the oral cavities, on the skin, and in the gut. They enter into the bloodstream through the gut and can travel to the joints.

And why is that a big deal?

Lipopolysaccharides (LPS), also known as a form of endotoxin, are like the waste products of certain 'bad' bacteria (gram-negative bacteria) that live in your gut. These waste products are normal. Usually, these stay within the confines of the gut and leave our body as waste, but sometimes they can escape into the bloodstream, particularly when the gut's lining lets more molecules into the bloodstream than it should or is damaged. Once in the bloodstream, LPS are considered foreign invaders and can trigger your body's immune system into action to fight invaders and protect itself. Small amounts don't seem to be a big problem for the body, but if there are more invaders than it can handle, or if the body's immune system is compromised due to other factors, then LPS can end up in different areas of the body, including the joints. That process can contribute to systemic inflammation in the body in general, but also locally in organs (e.g., the brain) and in joints.

How LPS Moves from the Gut to the Joints and Muscles

Imagine your gut as a coffee filter. Under normal circumstances, it lets through only what you want—e.g., coffee—while keeping the grounds out. However, when the filter has holes or tears, things that should stay contained, like coffee grounds (or in the body's case, LPS) leak out.

Therefore, if the coffee filter isn't working properly, you may get grounds in your coffee cup. So, too, substances like LPS can leak out of the gut and into the bloodstream, travel around the body, and land in many areas, including muscles and joints. Alternatively, if your gut is letting too much through (molecules from foods that aren't meant to be there, or by-products of bacteria like LPS), this situation is often called 'leaky gut syndrome,' or medical professionals refer to it as 'increased intestinal permeability'.

Due to poor diet, medications, stress, or illness, a leaky gut can occur and create low-grade systemic inflammation (an intangible trigger). This can impact joint and muscle health.

Once too much LPS escapes into your bloodstream, it sounds an alarm to your body's immune system. Your body reacts by sending signals that cause inflammation as a defense mechanism. When there is too much LPS for the body to manage, or if there is so much LPS that the immune response continues in overdrive, trying to keep its negative effects at bay, this inflammation response can affect the body systemically.

Impact on the Joints

While there is evidence that LPS traveling to the brain can potentially be related to depression and anxiety, when LPS travels to the joints, this endotoxin can cause degeneration of the cartilage (arthritis) and other tissues resulting in swelling, pain, and discomfort. Think about how a bunch of rowdy, drug-infused teenagers (LPS) can cause damage to the inside of a vacant house (your joints).

This damage can occur if the patient is overweight or normal weight. We know that excess weight on the body usually is an indicator of excess inflammation, but it is often thought that the reason that the joints of overweight or obese individuals are painful is due to excess weight putting too much pressure on the joints. This may only be partially true, as there are many overweight individuals who do not have joint pain, and many normal or underweight individuals who have arthritis and pain.

Research shows that if a person who is overweight or obese loses weight, this weight loss can improve the diversity of the gut and decrease intestinal permeability (leaky gut). This would, in turn, decrease how much LPS is entering the body and, subsequently, the joint, in addition to decreasing pressure on the joint.

Normal or underweight individuals can also improve the diversity of the gut through lifestyle and eating plan changes, thereby decreasing excessive intestinal permeability, and in turn, decreasing LPS in their joints.

Why One Joint and Not the Other?

Several patients over the years have had great questions about how the gut can impact joints, but one question always made me scratch my head.

Patients often asked, "Why would I have pain in one joint and not the other?"

After I had my anterior cruciate ligament (ACL) replaced following a college basketball injury, I was told by the doctor in 1986 that I would probably develop arthritis in that knee when I got older. I never understood why that would happen if they fixed it, but his prediction proved to be correct. However, as I explained earlier, I never had pain in the knee that had surgery until I injured it on the dance floor at a wedding. It was then, after an X-ray, that I discovered that I had a significant amount of arthritis in the joint that was 'fixed' four decades before. My opposite knee is perfectly fine: no pain and no signs of arthritis. So why did my surgical knee develop arthritis, even though the joint should have been as good as new after the surgery?

One study may have the answer. Researchers injected one group of mice with LPS and one group of mice with a saline solution five days prior to the mouse sustaining an ACL tear to one knee. When they assessed the tissue of the mice later, they found that the levels of osteoarthritis were slightly elevated in the female mice who had the saline injection, and not at all elevated in the males who had the same. But in the mice who had the LPS injection, the osteoarthritis that had developed in the injured joint was four to five times higher in the male mice, and four to six times higher in the female mice. So elevated levels of systemic LPS can potentially set someone up to develop arthritis in the joint or tissue that was injured or repaired surgically.

This would more than likely be true for my situation. In college, as an athlete that worked out two to three hours per day, sometimes twice a day, we often ate and drank what we wanted, and back in the day, it wasn't all vegetables and fruit. The carb avoidance phase was not on our radar at all. Add alcohol into the mix on the weekends along with a personal history of constipation, and I am sure my levels of LPS were elevated prior to the time that I injured my knee. The subsequent surgery I had contributed to additional trauma to the knee, and my healthy lifestyle changes did not kick in until more than a decade later after having my son and subsequent health problems. Therefore, it's plausible that is how my surgical knee developed a significant amount of arthritis and inflammation compared to the uninjured side that is free from any inflammation.

Lipopolysaccharide Impact on Muscles

Although research in this area is still emerging, evidence suggests that LPS can effect both smooth muscles (muscles we typically don't think about moving, e.g., the muscles of our bladder and our heart) and skeletal muscles (muscles that are typically under our conscious control, e.g., biceps, hamstrings, calves, etc.).

When women in one small study who were diagnosed with fibromyalgia (FM), a disorder that effects the muscles of the body, were injected with low levels of LPS, the women with fibromyalgia exhibited increased levels of pro-inflammatory responses and decreased anti-inflammatory responses compared to the control group injected with the same low levels of LPS.

Perhaps the levels of LPS were already elevated in the women with FM, since there is significant research about dysbiosis (poor gut health) in those with FM. This could be the reason for their excessive reaction to the endotoxin. Or those with FM may have a poorer response to inflammation in general.

In addition, a systemic review was able to assess the reaction of ninety-eight healthy subjects who received low dose injections of LPS. All of the participants had a lower pain threshold, meaning those who received the injection had a higher pain response (they felt the pain more) when muscle points were palpated after having the injection, in comparison to others who did not receive the injection. This indicated that increased LPS in the system can increase musculoskeletal pain sensitivity. Therefore, this leads researchers to believe there is yet another system the gut impacts: the gut-muscle axis. Let's add it to the list.

- The brain (gut-brain axis)
- The liver (gut-liver axis)
- The skin (gut-skin axis)
- The lungs (gut-lung axis)
- The kidneys (gut-kidney axis)
- The heart (gut-heart axis)
- The joints (gut-joint axis)
- The muscles (gut-muscle axis)

Therefore, chronic muscle pain with or without an injury could be due to excessive LPS in the system, caused by leaky gut, i.e., increased intestinal permeability.

What Can We Do About LPS?

If LPS and leaky gut is the problem, how do we stop LPS from escaping from the gut into the body and affecting our joints?

The process is similar to addressing a tangible trigger. When there is localized inflammation, such as after an injury to a joint, the best way to get rid of the inflammation is identify the trigger and remove it.

You may remember the plantar fasciitis that I experienced after I was walking differently, secondary to the knee injury that I had sustained a year prior. My hip was tight, and the change in the biomechanics in my knee from the injury resulted in a change in the biomechanics of my foot. This caused my arch to fall in more than usual (overpronation) and the excess stress that resulted on the plantar fascia of that foot ended up playing tug o' war with my heel. This resulted in pain.

Once I stretched my hip and strengthened it, along with the muscles supporting my knee, and addressed the issue with my arch, the pain went away. I followed these three steps:

Step 1) Find the trigger(s)
Step 2) Remove the trigger(s)
Step 3) Once the trigger(s) is/are eliminated, give the body what it needs to heal

So, how do we remove or decrease LPS if it's a trigger?

LPS Are Attached To Bacteria: Are Antibiotics The Answer?

LPS is a potential trigger. It's a major component of a 'bad' gram-negative bacteria. So, one might think antibiotics could be an answer since they are used to address bacterial infections. There are antibiotics that have been shown to lower LPS, like Colistin for example, but there doesn't appear to be any evidence that this medication or any other would be effective for osteoarthritis. Unfortunately, Colistin and other antibiotics have succumbed to antibiotic resistance. This occurs when the bacteria that the antibiotic has been able to kill has morphed into a more resistant bacteria against which the antibiotic is no longer effective.

At the time of this writing, there doesn't appear to be a commercially available prescription medication, either oral or injectable, that promises to lower the LPS or fix leaky gut associated with inflammation in joints and muscle without potentially creating more problems in the long-term.

How Do You Eliminate LPS in the Joints or Muscles?

Remember Jean, the volleyball fan? After doing SoftWave and addressing the localized inflammation in her knee, she was at a standstill. She was at the point where the treatment for localized inflammation in her knee wasn't getting her the sustained relief that we had hoped for.

I never want a patient to keep paying for visits if they aren't getting the results they seek. In our conversation, I looked back at Jean's initial consultation, and it was evident that she had issues with her gut along with a history of prediabetes. Prediabetes means that if Jean's blood sugar levels kept rising, she would eventually develop diabetes and have to take medications to control it.

She also had issues with bloating, constipation, and sometimes loose bowel movements. Jean started with a food and symptom diary. I asked her to keep track of the symptoms she experienced each day for two weeks so we could see if there were any correlations between what she was eating or drinking and the pain in her knee.

When Jean came back, we reviewed her food diary and the symptoms that she experienced.

After she filled this out, we learned quite a few things.

"What was your biggest takeaway from doing the food diary?" I asked Jean.

"Hmm, well, I know I don't eat enough fruits and vegetables," she replied.

"Okay, anything else?"

"I guess I also noticed that my knee felt worse on days that I ate poorly."

This was news to Jean. She really thought that her knee hurt all the time, but when she looked at her eating plan and when her knee pain was worse, there was definitely a difference on days she ate more processed and fast foods.

Looking at her food diary, we were able to see that the aching in her knee joint while she was trying to fall asleep was definitely worse after she had gone through the drive-thru of her local fast-food place or if she drank more alcohol than she normally did.

Next, I looked at how many of the foods that often cause inflammation in the body were regularly in Jean's diet. These foods are typically:

- Gluten-containing foods (think breads, baked goods, pastas, and packaged and processed foods)
- Processed foods with sugar (think sweets, baked goods, and bars)
- Dairy (think animal milk, cheese, and yogurt)

There was no doubt about it. In Jean's daily eating plan, almost every meal contained gluten.

"See here," I said as I circled all the gluten containing foods, "in pretty much every meal you have something that contains gluten."

Jean leaned in and nodded. "Okay, all those foods have gluten in them?"

"Yes."

Her eyes moved from the paper and back up to meet mine. "What is gluten anyway, and why is it a big deal?" she asked.

Gluten is a family of proteins found primarily in wheat, barley, and rye. It's what gives dough its elasticity and baked goods their chewy texture. When gluten-containing flour is mixed with water, the gluten proteins form a sticky network that has a glue-like consistency, which is why it's called "gluten," from the Latin word for glue.

Common foods that contain gluten include:

- Breads and pastries
- Pasta
- Cereals
- Beer
- Gravies and sauces (often thickened with flour)
- Processed or flavored snack foods, such as chips (sometimes) and pretzels
- Sushi (gluten makes the rice stick together)

"Is that what people with celiac disease have to avoid?" Jean asked.

"Yes, that is correct," I responded.

"I don't have celiac disease," said Jean. "I was tested for it before, because of my constipation, and they said it was negative."

"Even if a person does not have celiac disease, some people are still sensitive to gluten. This is called non-celiac gluten sensitivity (NCGS). It is a common digestive issue that affects people around the world. Our gut contains a complex community of bacteria, most of which are beneficial and necessary for our well-being. Sometimes, however, the balance of these bacteria can shift unfavorably—a condition called 'dysbiosis'—where harmful bacteria outnumber the beneficial ones, disrupting our body's normal functions. This imbalance can lead to inflammation in the gut, which manifests as symptoms like diarrhea, constipation, stomach pain, and general discomfort.

"In those with NCGS, this imbalance may also impact the communication between the gut, and the joints and muscles. That is, the gut-joint axis and the gut-muscle axis. This disruption can lead to increased inflammation both in the gut and throughout the body. One of the culprits that creates havoc when in excess in the body is lipopolysaccharide (LPS), a component of bacteria produced as the waste products of these harmful bacteria. LPS triggers inflammation in the body, including the joints, and it stimulates toll-like receptor 4, a part of the cell that is turned up when there is degeneration or breakdown of the tissue.

"In addition, people with NCGS can have other habits or conditions that can exacerbate their symptoms, including frequent alcohol consumption, regular use of anti-inflammatory drugs, a high-fat diet, or medical disorders such as diabetes, autoimmune issues, and fatty liver disease. These factors can intensify the symptoms of NCGS."

Jean sat back in her seat. "I've used a lot of anti-inflammatory medications to try and get rid of this pain for years."

"Yes, most of the patients I see with long-term issues have done the same."

"Could eating gluten be why I can't lose weight?"

"Many of the foods you are eating that contain gluten are processed, and mostly carbohydrates. These types of foods may not only be contributing to poor gut health and joint pain, but they could also be why you haven't lost more weight and still remain prediabetic."

"Man, really? So I have to get rid of all those foods?" Jean asked, pointing to the several circles I made on her food diary.

"If you want to start decreasing inflammation and improving your joint pain further, as well as help to regulate your blood sugar, avoid full-blown diabetes, and lose weight, then yes, gradually."

Jean stared at me in disbelief.

"You can start slow and begin replacing them one by one," I explained.

"I don't know if I can do that. What am I going to eat?"

Gluten-containing foods are very common in the American diet, largely due to the widespread use of wheat, barley, and rye in various products. Here are some of the main ways gluten is present in typical American meals:

- Bread and Baked Goods: Wheat flour, which contains gluten, is the primary ingredient in most bread, bagels, muffins, pastries, and cakes.
- Pasta and Noodles: Traditional pasta and noodles are typically made from wheat.
- Cereals: Many breakfast cereals are made from wheat, barley, and rye, or may contain malt flavoring, which is derived from barley.
- Snack Foods: Crackers, pretzels, cookies, and many other processed snacks often contain gluten.
- Processed Meats: Some sausages, hot dogs, and deli meats can contain gluten as a binder or filler.
- Sauces and Gravies: Wheat flour is a common thickener in many sauces and gravies.
- Beer and Malt Beverages: These typically contain barley malt.
- Ready Meals and Soups: Many pre-prepared dishes and soups use ingredients containing gluten.

Is Gluten Always the Problem?

Some of you may already have given up gluten but you still have joint pain. So, no, gluten isn't always the problem.

Jim never ate gluten.

"I can't eat bread and pasta; it kills my stomach. I even gave up beer, and only drink Tito's vodka now since it doesn't seem to make me feel as bad the next day."

This was Jim's response when I asked him about his diet. So, despite not eating gluten at all, Jim still had persistent back and hip pain. You met Jim in the introduction to this chapter.

He had fantastic results when we first started SoftWave. His pain went down to zero for several days at a time after the first and second treatments. But then it came back, though not as bad, and Jim was still frustrated.

"I really thought this was the answer," Jim told me as he shook his head.

"SoftWave is still part of the answer, Jim," I responded. "You have been having great results and you aren't in as much pain as when you came in."

"Yeah, well, what do we do now?"

"From here, we look at other factors that could be contributing to your pain. Let's talk about your eating plan."

"I already told you; I don't eat bread and all that other garbage."

"I understand, so we need to see what else could be contributing to your issue."

When I asked Jim to do a food and symptom diary, you would have thought I was asking him to climb Mount Everest backward. But I have to hand it to him, Jim arrived at his next session and pulled out a crumpled piece of paper and tossed it on my desk.

Highly Inflammatory Foods

"That's the best I could do."

"Thanks, Jim!" I said smiling as I smoothed out the crinkled sheet.

I asked Jim what he learned, and as he looked away from my eye contact, he replied, "Nothing, that's what I'm paying you for."

"Okay, here we go." I got out my blue pen and methodically went through his food diary as well as his symptoms.

"So, Jim, on this day, you rated your pain a two out of ten, and then four days later, it was up to a seven. Did you notice that?"

"Yeah, I wrote it down, didn't I?" he replied in obvious annoyance.

"You sure did. What's the biggest difference here between this day and the rest?"

"We went up north," he said.

"It looks like you had some wine and a few other alcoholic beverages. Lots of cheese and sausage with gluten-free crackers on the days when your pain increased."

"Yep, we do live in Wisconsin, you know."

"Yes, I am aware Jim, I'm aware," I said with a smirk.

"What's the big deal with red meat and alcohol anyway?" Jim waved at the piece of paper in front of me. "I don't have them all the time."

Not everyone has issues with these foods, but I shared with Jim a few reasons why some people do.

Red Meat

- High in Purines: Red meat contains high levels of purines, which the body metabolizes into uric acid. Elevated levels of uric acid from excess consumption of red meat can lead to the formation of crystals in the joints, causing painful inflammation typical of gout.

- Arachidonic Acid: This type of fatty acid found in red meat can be converted into prostaglandins, which are inflammatory compounds. These prostaglandins can exacerbate inflammation in the joints.
- Saturated Fat: The high content of saturated fats in red meat can increase inflammation throughout the body. Chronic inflammation is a key factor in many types of joint pain and arthritis.
- Gut Dysbiosis and Permeability: Diets high in red meat can alter the gut microbiota and increase gut permeability, often referred to as "leaky gut." This condition can allow more LPS to pass from the gut into the bloodstream, enhancing systemic inflammation.

Alcohol

- Uric Acid Production: The metabolism of alcohol can lead to increased production and decreased excretion of uric acid, thus raising its levels in the blood and potentially causing gout attacks.
- Increases Inflammation: Alcohol consumption boosts the production of inflammatory molecules and reduces the liver's ability to clear these and other inflammatory substances, including LPS, from the bloodstream.
- Gut Permeability: Alcohol damages the gut lining, enhancing its permeability and allowing substances like LPS to enter the bloodstream more easily. This increases systemic inflammation.
- Impaired Liver Function: Chronic alcohol use can impair liver function, further hampering the body's ability to filter out LPS and other toxins, which contributes to systemic inflammation.

"But I've eaten these foods all my life and never had an issue before."

"How long has your back and hip been bothering you?" I asked.

"A long time." Jim's gaze moved up toward the ceiling. "I mean, probably ten years. But it's just recently gotten worse."

"There are a few reasons that your body may be reacting to these foods more now than before. Let's walk through some of them . . ."

1. Cumulative Effects

- **Uric Acid Accumulation**: Regular consumption of high-purine foods (like red meat) and alcohol can lead to a gradual build-up of uric acid over time. After passing through the liver, most of the uric acid is excreted in urine or through the intestines. The kidneys remove two-thirds of uric acid, and the GI tract removes the other third. If these systems gradually slow down, it may take years for uric acid levels to reach a point where they cause gout or other forms of joint pain.
- **Inflammatory Load**: Both red meat (due to saturated fats and other inflammatory agents) and alcohol can contribute to systemic inflammation. The liver and spleen are the primary filters for removing LPS and other inflammatory molecules from the blood, with the majority of elimination being through the liver. As we age, if these organ systems become sluggish in their filtering system due to medications, lack of micronutrients, or stress, inflammation throughout the body can increase. Chronic, low-level inflammation can slowly damage joint tissues, with symptoms becoming noticeable only after the development of significant damage.

2. Aging and Decreased Kidney Function

- As people age, their kidney function often declines. This reduction in renal efficiency can lead to decreased clearance of uric acid from the body, raising its levels in the blood and potentially leading to gout or other forms of joint pain.

3. Weight Gain

- Long-term consumption of calorie-dense foods like red meat and alcoholic beverages can lead to weight gain. Increased body weight puts additional stress on the joints, particularly weight-bearing ones like the knees and hips, which can exacerbate joint pain and problems. As we previously discussed, habits can also increase LPS, which is related to degeneration in joints.

4. Development of Comorbid Conditions

- Over time, other health conditions such as diabetes, hypertension, or hyperlipidemia may develop, which can complicate and exacerbate joint issues. These conditions can also contribute to systemic inflammation and poorer overall health, impacting joints.

5. Tolerance and Thresholds

- The body can sometimes adapt to certain levels of toxins or stressors (like uric acid and inflammation) up to a point. Over time, as the burden increases or the body's adaptive capacity declines, symptoms may emerge as the body can no longer compensate.

6. Behavioral Changes

- Changes in activity levels or diet (even if not recognized) can also tip the balance, exacerbating symptoms that were previously minor or unnoticed.

7. Increased Sensitivity

- Finally, joints may become more sensitive due to wear and tear, previous minor injuries, or reduced repair capacity, making them more susceptible to problems from dietary sources.

"So, as you can see, Jim, the red meat and certain types of alcohol could be contributing to that low-grade inflammation over time and the potentially increased LPS in the body, causing the joint pain to come and go."

"Do I have to give up all of it?" Jim asked.

Elimination Diet

Neither Jean nor Jim was excited to make the dietary changes I recommended, but the pain was bad enough that they were willing to give it their best shot. After all, both had improvements on our program, whereas other programs and treatments provided little to no relief.

It took a while for Jean to find gluten-free alternatives to the foods she was used to eating. Instead of getting rid of everything processed, she looked for treats that she could have that were gluten-free. The challenge, though, with many gluten-free foods is there are more sugars and additives in them. Baked goods that are gluten-free often have a significant amount of sugar, chemicals as sugar substitutes, and fats. But she found that if she limited these processed gluten-free foods, she could manage her blood sugars better. The rest of the time, she was eating healthy, unprocessed food such as vegetables, some fruit, good fat, and protein. She added nuts to her diet as well for a healthy snack.

But the real test was yet to come. Her trip to Disneyland with her family was coming up, and it was the catalyst for her jumping into gluten-free eating. She wanted to enjoy this time and not spend it on the sidelines wishing she could participate in the fun.

Honestly, I was pretty nervous myself. We only had six or seven weeks prior to her trip to get her eating plan to the point where she was experiencing decreased pain in her knee. I pulled out all the stops. We found the best and most supportive knee brace. She had comfortable inserts in her newly broken-in walking shoes. I taught her how to strap her knee with Kinesio tape to take some pressure off her kneecap. We discussed how she could ice, keep compression on her knee, and when not walking around, keep it elevated. She restarted her SoftWave sessions because they started to bring her more relief, likely due to less inflammation in her entire system.

With each passing week, Jean reported less pain in her knee, less fluid around her body, improved digestion, weight loss, and better blood sugar readings.

Three weeks had passed since Jean's last appointment when I saw her name pop up on my schedule. I felt my stomach do a flip-flop.

- What if all the work we had done to get her knee feeling better was totally reversed when she did all that walking in Disneyland?
- What if she reverted to eating all the processed foods so readily available at the amusement park and that flared her up?
- What if she ended up having a miserable time? After all, I was the one encouraging her all along to stick with it since she was seeing so much benefit before she left.

My chest rose and fell sharply a few times as Jean entered the room. I detected a slight limp, though it was much better than previous times.

"Come on in, traveler," I said, trying to keep the conversation light. "How are you? How did it go?" I noticed my voice sounded higher than usual.

Jean sat in front of me, and slowly but surely her mouth morphed into a huge smile. "I did great," she replied, her eyes beamed. "It was such a good trip."

I leaned in and laid my hands flat on the desk. "Tell me all about it."

Jean went on to tell me that she was able to pack a cooler with all of her gluten-free food and keep it in her car. They would leave the park occasionally to go have their snacks. Her husband was happy to do it, since it ended up saving them a significant amount of money not eating the overpriced park food. Her daughter was annoyed to have to leave the park at times, but overall, she was thrilled that Jean could go on all the rides and walk for hours. And best of all, Jean said, "My knee felt great."

I couldn't have been happier for her.

When Food Fuels Pain

Jim struggled for quite a few weeks to give up the red meat and alcohol.

"It was harder than I thought," he complained.

But eventually, he admitted, on the days he avoided those foods and drinks, his back and hip felt so much better.

"The relief did not happen right away, though," Jim explained. "Sometimes it was like my joints had a hangover from too much red meat and alcohol."

He went on to report that it would take a couple of days for his back and hip to feel better, once he abstained from both.

I noticed Jim's typically red and inflamed cheeks started to fade to a more normal, fair complexion.

He wouldn't commit to sticking to this new diet forever, but he finally did admit that he believed changing his diet was a game-changer for his joint pain.

How can I explain the significant improvement in Jean and Jim's symptoms?

Because there aren't any reliable over-the-counter blood tests yet to determine if lipopolysaccharides had indeed decreased and systemic inflammation subsided, and physicians do not normally do any of the tests available to assess if the gut is leaky or has increased permeability, I can't say for sure that is what happened. But the significant symptom reduction in the previously painful joints, plus the additional improvements that both Jean and Jim experienced with their gut health, weight, and skin lead me to believe their bodies were doing what they instinctively want to do for all of us ... they want to heal. Taking away these tangible triggers like gluten for Jean and red meat and alcohol for Jim likely led to intangible triggers like LPS and systemic inflammation subsiding and allowed the inflammatory cycle to go about its merry way to resolve some inflammation, and, in turn, decrease symptoms.

Tests To Determine Leaky Gut or Presence of LPS in the Body

I haven't ever witnessed physicians ordering the following tests for leaky gut, LPS, or increased intestinal permeability, but according to the Cleveland Clinic, these are tests under investigation:

- Urine Test: You drink a special drink with different types of sugars. Some of these sugars typically don't get absorbed by your intestines. Later, your urine is tested to see which sugars passed through your gut.
- Blood Test: A sample of your blood is checked for signs of gut bacteria. Scientists look for certain things in your blood, like antibodies and toxins. One test for LPS is not commonly available right now.
- Tissue Biopsy: In this more invasive test, a small piece of your intestine is examined. Scientists use electricity to measure how well ions (small particles) move across your gut lining into the bloodstream.
- Confocal Endomicroscopy: This advanced test lets doctors see your gut lining up close and in detail. They use a special dye that, if there are gaps in your gut lining, will show up in your intestines.

My hope is that someday we will be able to reliably measure lipopolysaccharides and leaky gut in a way that we can see exactly what someone needs to improve their gut health. But for now, the formula that I typically use to help my patients is, as you know, find the trigger and remove it, but also give the gut what it needs to recondition itself.

Gut Reconditioning

In addition to optimizing their eating plan, we introduced Jean and Jim to our gut reconditioning program to help the body initiate its own healing process. This consists of:

- A good quality probiotic
- A fiber-rich supplement with herbal support for elimination and gut repair
- A soothing blend of herbs that help to encourage natural mucus production in the gut and naturally decrease inflammation

These supplements are added to their program. Over the years, anecdotally, I have seen great results related to optimizing gut health when patients utilize this program. We will discuss how this program works in the next chapter.

Bonus Material
JOINT PAIN AND CHANGES IN WEATHER

If I had a dollar for every patient over the last few decades who told me they felt like they could forecast the weather changes by the pain in their joints, I would most definitely be retired by now.

When it comes to pain in joints and rainy weather, the role of barometric pressure cannot be ignored. Though researchers will try to tell you it doesn't make any difference, my patients tell me a completely different story. Take eighty-two-year-old Barbara. She can predict an upcoming rainstorm with amazing accuracy just by the way her knee and shoulder feel a few days before a storm. She is not alone. Whenever I hear a patient complaining about this, I automatically talk to them about their gut health, and most times they think I'm crazy.

But hear me out. Barometric pressure, also known as atmospheric pressure, is the weight of the atmosphere pressing down on the Earth's surface. It fluctuates with weather changes and can significantly affect our joints.

As a storm approaches, barometric pressure typically drops. This decrease in pressure affects joints, especially for those with pre-existing conditions such as osteoarthritis or rheumatoid arthritis. Some joints like the knee, shoulder, hip, ankle, and even the joints of the spine contain synovial fluid, which serves as a lubricant and cushion and makes these joints susceptible to changes in the barometric pressure. These changes in weather can cause the tissues around the joints to expand or contract slightly, influencing the pressure within the joint.

Consequently, this can lead to heightened pressure and discomfort, resulting in joint pain during rainy weather.

As we strive to understand the complex relationship between weather and joint pain, an emerging concept deserves attention—the connection between gut health and joint pain during weather changes. Recent research has introduced the intriguing hypothesis that links gut health to joint pain during changes in barometric pressure.

Leaky gut, medically known as increased intestinal permeability, as discussed, is a condition where the lining of the intestines becomes more porous, allowing substances to pass through more easily. It has been associated with various health issues, including autoimmune diseases and joint pain. You now understand that research has shown that an imbalance in gut microbiota and inflammation can contribute to leaky gut.

How Leaky Gut Relates to Weather-Induced Joint Pain

The connection between leaky gut and weather-induced joint pain begins to take shape when we consider the impact of falling barometric pressure on the gut. According to Boyle's law, "decreased barometric pressure causes the intestinal gas volume to expand." (Yamamoto, 2020).

Excess gas in the intestines may contribute to increased gut inflammation and further compromise the integrity of the intestinal barrier. If leaky gut is exacerbated during weather changes, it could allow more bacteria like LPS and other toxins to migrate from the gut into the bloodstream. This, in turn, could lead to systemic and localized inflammation, potentially affecting the joints.

It's important to emphasize that this theory is still in the realm of emerging research. Studies are needed to confirm these connections definitively. However, it offers a novel perspective on why some individuals experience heightened joint pain before storms.

In the clinical setting, I have noticed that people who have aching in their joints when the weather changes often have less than optimal diet, gut issues, or only short-term relief with our SoftWave device. This is a strong indication that the problem with joint pain is potentially coming from the gut.

Key Pieces

Gut-Joint Axis and Gut-Muscle Axis: The gut and joints as well as

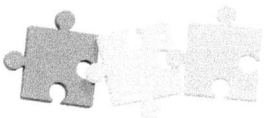

muscles are intricately connected through the gut-joint and gut-muscle axis. These axes give an example of how the gut microbiota plays a significant role in regulating inflammation that can impact joint and muscle health.

Lipopolysaccharides (LPS): LPS, a bacterial endotoxin found in the gut, can escape into the bloodstream through a 'leaky gut,' leading to systemic inflammation that affects joints and muscles, potentially worsening conditions like osteoarthritis and fibromyalgia.

Diet and Inflammation: Some foods can exacerbate gut dysbiosis and increase intestinal permeability, leading to greater LPS levels and inflammation in the joints.

Personalized Treatment: Addressing gut health through dietary changes, like reducing or eliminating inflammatory foods, can significantly alleviate joint and muscle pain, as demonstrated by case studies involving patients like Jean and Jim.

Barometric Pressure and Joint Pain: Weather changes, particularly decreases in barometric pressure, may exacerbate joint pain in individuals with leaky gut by increasing gut inflammation and LPS migration into the bloodstream.

Want to dig a little deeper?
Go to https://newyouhealthandwellness.com/ebooks/ to find out more about how to address your gut health to get rid of muscle and joint pain and watch our gut health joint health video at https://newyouhealthandwellness.com/what-is-the-gut-joint-axis/

CHAPTER 10
When Good Food is Bad for You

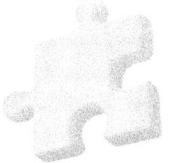

"Let food be thy medicine and medicine be thy food."

–Hippocrates

As dawn crept over the horizon, my fingers curled around the typically warm steering wheel as I headed to work. This normally sent a gentle sense of comfort through my system, but for several weeks, these fingers had already been protesting the morning ritual with a dull, persistent throb in each joint. Each twist of the wheel was a chore, while pangs rotating from aching to stiffness radiated from the joints like reluctant whispers from a bunch of rusty hinges. With every stoplight or sign, I closed and opened my fists, followed by fervently shaking them in mid-air. At times, the pain made the simple act of driving feel like navigating through a bramble of thorns. By the time late morning came around, typically the pain was gone.

That was my life for a few months, and I couldn't figure out why.

I had already been off gluten due to my back and leg pain disappearing after I stopped including it in my diet.

Seriously, I have barely had dairy and have recently lost weight by minimizing sugar. What do I have to change now? I thought.

After X-rays that revealed normal healthy joints, and since there was no injury that I remembered, I felt frustrated that I had been working so hard to remain healthy by being active and eating right, yet now I had this pain. Its relentless irritation motivated me to find a solution.

Doing the Best She Could

When Kelly came to see me, she was equally frustrated. On her first visit, she slumped into the chair across from me, her face etched with the lines of fatigue and frustration that only relentless discomfort could draw. She reported feeling achy all over, tired, and irritated that despite her efforts at nourishing her body with clean, wholesome foods, the stubborn scale refused to move in her favor. With each tired blink and polite, strained smile, Kelly's weariness seeped into the space between us, palpable and poignant.

"I truly don't know what else to do," she said. "No matter what, whether I exercise or not, whether I eat more or less, I can't lose weight, and I just don't feel any better!"

Normally, if Kelly had come to see me with complaints of one or two joints hurting, I would have taken her through a biomechanical evaluation, but her symptoms were diffuse and not a result of any specific injury. At this point, I usually consider whether hormones or her gut health and eating plan could be the cause, and with further discussion, it became apparent which area we needed to assess first.

"This must be so frustrating. I see on your consultation sheet that you have some digestive issues. Can you give me some more detail about those symptoms?"

Kelly went on to describe that she felt bloated and uncomfortable most of the time, no matter what she ate. "The symptoms did improve when I changed my diet, but I still have discomfort and trouble going to the bathroom."

As I looked across the table and listened intently, I couldn't help but think about the symptoms I, myself, had experienced years before. Despite doing everything right and eating an anti-inflammatory diet, I had still been experiencing pain. Lucky for me, my symptoms were localized to my hands, and I wasn't currently experiencing the relentless fatigue Kelly was having. Due to her achy joints and general discomfort, I was confident that when she started our program, her joint pain and her fatigue could improve.

Food Sensitivities Testing

I tend to be a big-time skeptic, never fully believing that something is going to work just because one other person had a positive experience or one study showed a certain outcome. It takes a lot of research and my own experiences, as well as the experiences of others for me to jump on board and recommend a treatment for my patients.

I have learned to be more open-minded than I was in my youth, realizing that going through conventional training for my Bachelor of Science back in the late 1980s resulted in an unconscious bias toward anything considered unconventional. But I was even skeptical of medications, which I tended to shy away from anyway. For something to convince me, it had to be proven scientifically, or at the least make sense based on the basic anatomy, physiology, and movement science that I was exposed to in my undergraduate degree. Where I earned my degree, there was both an undertone and an obvious bias that many of my professors, and certainly the textbooks I was reading, displayed against anything 'natural' or complimentary. They were often completely against 'natural' remedies, classifying them as "snake oil." Any testing not prescribed by a physician, which at that time was pretty much everything except for blood tests, X-rays, and MRI, were considered irrelevant and unreliable.

But as I matured, through my own experience and the experience I had with patients, I saw that not all patients responded the way they were supposed to. It was often very tempting to explain poor results away as:

- The patient being noncompliant
- Not doing their exercises at all or enough
- Not taking the advice we gave them about better supportive shoes, particular exercises, following up with ergonomic changes at their desk to help relieve shoulder and neck pain, or the best way to sleep with certain pillows to help their neck or back

Their lack of compliance was always the easy excuse for lack of outcomes. I couldn't help but wonder why some patients who swore up and down that they were doing everything right just weren't getting better.

And then it happened to me.

My hands started aching every day on the way to work, as I described earlier in the chapter. But also, at the same time, I had a patient who had celiac disease. She mentioned to me that her joints had been extremely sore before they diagnosed her with celiac disease, and when she came off the gluten, the aching in her joints went away. I confirmed by reviewing research about celiac disease that, in fact, joint pain was a symptom. When contemplating my own situation, I knew that I had been off gluten for several years, so my hand pain couldn't be due to gluten. At that moment, a proverbial light bulb went off over my head.

What if there were other types of foods that could cause joint pain? I dug into the research and stumbled upon something called "food sensitivities."

I had heard of food allergies before. I had heard of food intolerances. But I had never heard of food sensitivities.

For the purpose of this book, and since there are several different definitions of food intolerance or insensitivity, we are defining food allergies and food intolerance according to the American Academy of Allergy, Asthma, and Immunology (AAAAI) and food sensitivities as the following:

Food Allergy

- Definition: According to the AAAAI, food allergy is an immune system reaction that occurs soon after eating a specific food. Even a tiny amount of the allergy-causing food can trigger signs and symptoms such as digestive problems, hives, or swollen airways. In some cases, a food allergy can cause severe symptoms or even a life-threatening reaction known as anaphylaxis.
- Key Characteristics: Involves the immune system, particularly the IgE antibodies. Symptoms are often more severe and can be life-threatening.

Food Intolerance

- Definition: According to the AAAAI, food intolerance refers to difficulty digesting certain foods and having an unpleasant physical reaction to them. It does not involve the immune system. Symptoms are generally less serious and often limited to digestive problems.
- Key Characteristics: Does not involve the immune system. Symptoms are primarily gastrointestinal and include bloating, gas, diarrhea, and stomach pain. It's often dose-dependent, meaning problems are worse with larger quantities of the offending food.

Food Sensitivity

- Definition: Food sensitivity is a broad term that includes any adverse reaction to food that does not fit the typical definitions of allergy or intolerance. It can involve various symptoms like headaches, joint pain, and fatigue, which are not always immediate and can vary in severity. This term is not generally accepted in the medical community.
- Key Characteristics: May involve different parts of the immune system and does not always have a clear mechanism. Symptoms can be wide-ranging, delayed, and are less predictable compared to allergies and intolerances.

Food sensitivities don't have an agreed-upon definition that is accepted by conventional medicine, so I am using the definition above to show you how I explain this to my patients.

In a nutshell, someone can be sensitive to a food, but the reaction from eating that food may not happen to the person until hours or days later, or in some cases, after several days of exposure to that food. The reaction may also be mild, and many times does not cause visible damage to the gut on inspection with a medical procedure, such as endoscopy, that puts a camera down your throat and passes through your stomach into the small intestine, or a colonoscopy that puts a camera up through the anal canal to inspect the lower part of the large intestine. My patients with gut issues that they feel are related to foods have had tests such as the endoscopy or colonoscopy, and no damage was reported. They often are told it's all in their head, or it's just due to stress. A frequent diagnosis for these people is irritable bowel syndrome (IBS).

Did you ever eat a meal and within an hour or two you were bloated, have gas, feel fatigued, experience brain fog, or have achy joints? Yeah, me too. This could be a food intolerance.

Celiac disease used to be considered a food intolerance until, according to the AAAAI, was determined that it is an autoimmune disease. Typically, I will still refer to it as an intolerance because those who have celiac disease are intolerant to gluten and must avoid it. If they ingest gluten, it will create significant damage to structures in the small intestine called villi. See Figure 10.1.

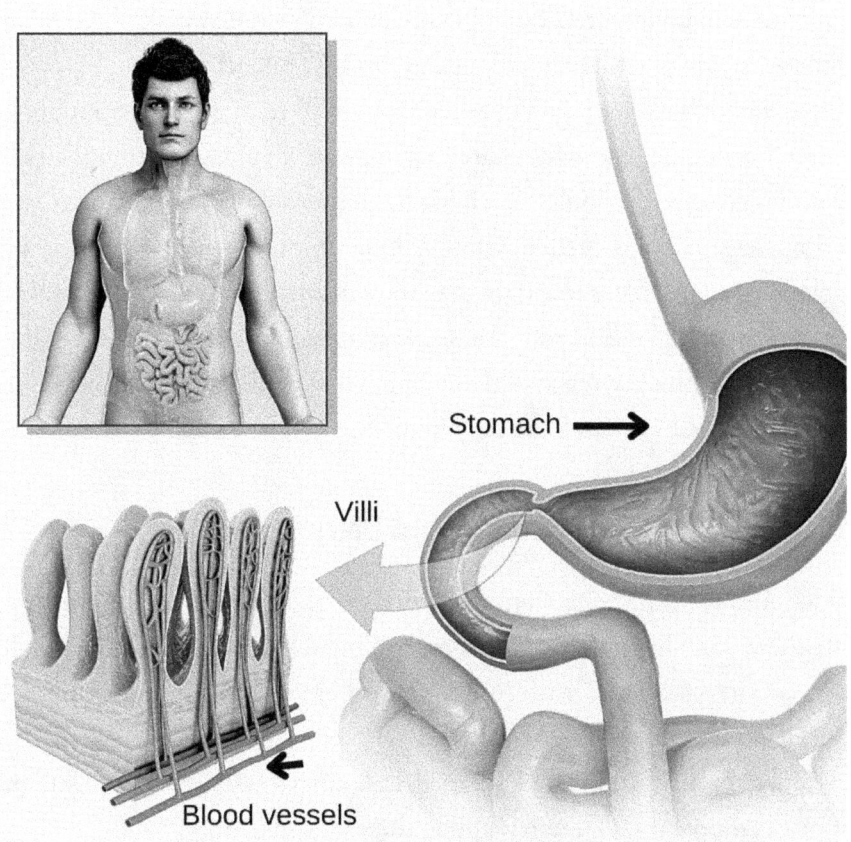

Figure 10.1 Villi from the small intestine

These structures in the gut help nutrients from food get absorbed into the bloodstream. Once in the bloodstream, these nutrients can travel where they are needed in the body. Damage to these structures eventually causes malnutrition in the patient, joint pain, inflammation, and fatigue, and some of these patients are diagnosed with other autoimmune diseases.

On the other hand, if you have a food allergy, you have an immediate immune reaction where, for example, you immediately break out in hives or worse, your airway could close up, and the event could be life-threatening. This is called anaphylaxis.

Food sensitivities can be implicated when symptoms don't show up right away after eating the offending foods. This made sense based on the patients that I had seen over the years who felt better after stopping gluten but hadn't reacted to gluten right away when having it in the past. At times symptoms would take hours or days to show up. Some patients did not even have digestive issues, but at times felt tired and generally unwell. It seemed like some days they were fine with gluten, and other days, not so much. But like in my case, some symptoms persisted, or new ones appeared despite staying away from gluten. Therefore, gluten-containing foods couldn't have been the only culprit.

What About Dairy?

It's common knowledge that some people react to the lactose in milk, but there can also be issues with a protein in dairy, i.e., whey or casein. This can be associated with inflammation in the gut, similar to that of gluten in those with Celiac disease.

Since neither Kelly nor I ate or drank dairy regularly, the frequency of our symptoms ruled dairy out as the cause of pain.

So, the question remained: were there other foods, even foods considered 'healthy' that impacted Kelly's gut and mine? Could these foods potentially trigger systemic inflammation? In my case, it might have been the gut-joint axis, and perhaps the gut-brain axis and gut-joint axis in Kelly's situation? If yes, how could this be happening?

Our Unique Microbiome

Since all of us have different physiologies and eat different foods, our gut bacteria is unique as a fingerprint. Research shows only 5 to 20 percent of our microbiome is the same as the next person. Could it be possible that each of us reacts differently to many different foods? Even foods that are considered healthy? If yes, how do we find out?

Food Sensitivity Testing

When I was weighing my options about which test to have done in order to find out why my hands started aching every morning, I knew I needed something other than a food allergy test. After all, I wasn't breaking out or having a significant reaction, such as my throat swelling, which could land me in the hospital. It was a good couple of hours between me leaving my house in the morning and having breakfast. I wondered if my smoothie was the culprit.

The typical smoothie for me during the time my hands started to hurt consisted of almond milk, greens (typically spinach), cashews or macadamias, my "green stuff" (a mix of powdered fruits and vegetables), protein powder (sometimes whey, sometimes rice bran), and some filtered water. I perfected the mix to my taste buds and felt amazing each morning after I had it, until one to two hours later when I got in the car.

As time went on, and I started to pay attention to the pain instead of choosing to ignore it, hoping it would eventually go away. And with the help of my food and symptom diary, I was able to narrow it down to my breakfast. But with all the variety of ingredients I would put in that smoothie, I wasn't excited to try eliminating one ingredient at a time to see which one may have been the culprit. The green powder I added had fifteen different vegetables and fruit, So that would be a long, frustrating, expensive experiment.

This is where my hunt for the best food sensitivity test began.

At first, I was drawn to companies that were offering IgG testing because, honestly, they were the cheapest option. But a few of my friends had them done and had varying results. One millennial noticed that eggs came up on her IgG food sensitivity test. She had always thought there was a dairy issue, but that came up normal. She got rid of the eggs and felt much better. That was an encouraging result, but nothing else came up for her. One couple did the IgG test and told me nothing came up for either of them. That was extremely odd. Everyone has some reaction to foods, even if it's just a normal mild reaction occasionally. They both had symptoms of chronic back pain that was resistant to any treatment, and one of them experienced constipation regularly, so their results surprised me.

I looked into IgG testing and found its results reflect exposure to a type of food rather than any adverse reaction. In other words, IgG testing may tell you what foods you are tolerant of or having frequently, but not what foods you are sensitive or intolerant to.

Then I came across the antigen leukocyte cellular antibody test, otherwise known as the ALCAT. It is specifically designed to uncover food sensitivities by looking at components of the immune system called white blood cells (or leukocytes) present in the blood. It measures response to foods, but if you would like, you can order testing for reactions to chemicals, herbs, molds, fungus, and other substances. The test is based on the premise that the reactions observed when exposing white blood cells (a marker of our immune system) to different foods, may correlate to symptoms such as bloating, constipation, diarrhea, but also skin irritation and inflammatory conditions such as irritable bowel syndrome, and from what I observe, muscle and joint pain.

Conventional medicine has had lackluster results from their own tradition of skin prick testing to assess food allergies. It is worth noting that traditional skin prick testing is accurate for food allergies 50 percent of the time. When conventional medicine practitioners put down other testing, saying theirs is the gold standard, they don't reveal that the 'gold standard' testing works half of the time.

Though the reliability of the ALCAT has been questioned by conventional medicine and by countless publications like the *New York Times*, touting lack of evidence, other research has been published supporting the ALCAT's reliability and validity.

The ALCAT has been found to have reproducibility, sensitivity, and specificity; the holy trinity related to solid research findings. Yale's findings endorsed the ALCAT's ability to identify foods that trigger inflammatory responses. Another research study in *Clinical Nutrition* in 2018 reported that the ALCAT can be a valuable test to determine non-celiac gluten sensitivity.

In a sea full of options, with price tags ranging from $50 to $1000, based on the research I reviewed, my decision was to get the blood test required for the ALCAT and make a commitment to follow through with my results.

The ALCAT Results

To say I was excited to get my ALCAT results back was an understatement. I wanted to know what I may have been reacting to in my smoothie, and these results were going to save me a lot of time and energy.

An email arrived in my inbox letting me know the results were in. I clicked on the pdf to find a very organized summary containing three columns of information.

One column had a red heading, the second column had an orange heading, and the third had a yellow one. These represented the specific foods I was reacting to severely, moderately, and minimally, respectively, when the immune cells from my blood were exposed to these foods. Next to these three columns was a column with a green heading. These are the foods I had no reaction to, and they were broken down into categories such as meats, fruits, vegetables, grains, etc.

And finally, on the bottom of the sheet there were four blue boxes. Each separate blue box represented whether I reacted to gluten, dairy, or sugary foods.

Even though I encourage my patients to always focus on all the options they did not have reactions to, my eyes were guilty of immediately scanning the severe and moderate columns. I finally found my offending food. Well, it's not the food's fault I guess, but I was surprised and relieved to have some hope of getting rid of my symptoms. As I stared at the paper, the word *spinach* jumped out at me. Guess what the base of my smoothies had been?

Yep, spinach.

I was trying to do the right thing and eat more plant-based foods. Spinach, though not able to compare to the amount of iron and protein in meats, is a good source of these nutrients for a plant. But I was reacting severely to it. My inner child wanted to call my mom and tell her that there clearly was a reason my body did not want to have that kind of slimy canned spinach growing up! I was vindicated at last. :)

The other ingredients in my morning smoothie were either nonreactive or minimally so. My experiment was to remove just one ingredient, i.e., Popeye's favorite snack, and see what happened to my hands. Sure enough, the next day I added arugula (from my green list) and there was no aching in my hands on the way to work. What a relief!

Why spinach? Great question. In my case, I believe I was overdoing spinach and having it on a regular basis in large quantities in my smoothies. Spinach, like other foods listed below, contains oxalates.

> Oxalates are naturally occurring compounds found in many foods, including leafy greens and berries. When oxalic acid combines with heavy metals or free minerals, it forms crystals that can deposit in soft tissues, joints, glands, and bones, causing chronic pain. Some foods that are high in oxalates include:
>
> - Nuts and seeds: Almonds, cashews, peanuts, sesame seeds, and chia seeds
> - Vegetables: Spinach, Swiss chard, zucchini, collard greens, celery, carrots, beets, berries, currants, and figs
> - Fruit: Kiwi, orange peel, raspberries, tangerine, and fruit cocktail
> - Other: Chocolate, beer, black tea, instant coffee, hot chocolate, soy drinks, wheat bran, grits, amaranth, buckwheat, cereal, fruit cake, pretzels, and whole wheat flour

Though spinach and possibly the oxalates were issues for me, they may not be an issue for you. The ALCAT helped me zero in on the food that wasn't agreeing with me and was contributing to my joint pain.

The Best Kind of Side Effect

Kelly's results were completely different than mine.

At her next appointment, I went on to explain the different columns and categories from her ALCAT report. She had been feeling slightly better since the first time we met, which I attributed to the bowel reconditioning program she started after her initial consultation (see Appendix for details). Some overall fatigue had lifted, but she was still a bit sore all over. Though she felt less bloated, the brain fog, general joint pain, and the excess weight and other symptoms still remained.

"Well, what do you think?" I asked Kelly.

"About the results? They are very interesting," she replied thoughtfully.

"Any deal breakers on there? Foods that you love and you don't think you could give up?"

"Not really. I mean, you said it was only for three to six months, right? Then I can start adding stuff back in?"

"Yes, that's right. You continue the bowel reconditioning program and cleanse to help with elimination, decreasing inflammation, and improving gut health. Then, after three months, you can add a food from the moderate category back in and see how you feel. Then after six months, you can add the one from your severe list that you really like."

"Do I have to add them back?"

"No, definitely not. Only if you want to."

"And why am I on this reconditioning program again?"

"The bowel reconditioning program is comprised of a good quality probiotic, a fiber supplement to help with elimination, and a combination of herbs that help support the production of healthy mucus and short-chained fatty acids in your bowel. The idea is to clean out your gut, sprinkle in the probiotic to help support your microbiome, and then utilize the mucilage herbs to help create healthy mucus to soothe and protect your gut."

"Is everyone's program the same?"

"Each person's is similar, but not always the same."

"How do you know this reconditioning works?" she asked.

"If you recall, we talked about a patient of mine in the past who had gone in to have an endoscopy after being on my program for about a year. Her first test showed there was damage that the doctor rated as an eight out of ten. And after she had the test redone, he wasn't able to detect damage at all. He said if he hadn't done the first test himself, he would have said she was misdiagnosed. That taught me that if we:

1. Remove the trigger causing the irritation and inflammation
2. Give the body the nutrients and nourishment it needs to heal
3. The body can carry out its innate healing ability on tissue that was once damaged

This helps to repair the gut lining, and potentially could decrease the molecules getting into the bloodstream that shouldn't be there, as well as bacteria such as LPS that can wreak havoc all around our body including the joints."

Kelly agreed to stick with the program, do another food diary for our next meeting, and put her health first.

I saw Kelly two to three times in the next six-to-eight-month period. And it was her third visit after our first meeting that was the most exciting.

Sitting across the desk from me was a new woman. Her face was thinning. Her eyes were brighter. She sat taller in her seat. And the smile beaming in my direction enveloped me.

"Kelly, you look great! How are you feeling?"

"So much better!"

She went on to tell me that her brain fog was gone. Her joint pain disappeared and she had lost an additional twenty-seven pounds despite being extremely busy at work and not having a lot of time for exercise. Not a bad side effect from getting rid of inflammatory foods.

Kelly stayed on the eating plan. And at the time of this writing, she has lost nearly fifty pounds. She now has energy and motivation to exercise. Her story is illustrated in our blog on an episode of our local morning show, *The Morning Blend*. (https://newyouhealthandwellness.com/morningblendepisodes/)

To date, any person who has been committed to making the adjustments with ALCAT and following our program as recommended has significantly reduced their joint and muscle pain, improved their energy levels, and many have lost weight to varying degrees. At times, for those who are normal weight, we have to add food to their eating plan so that they maintain a good healthy weight throughout.

There are foods that Kelly wasn't able to add back into her daily meal plans because she still felt that she reacted to them, but in Kelly's words, "Why would I add those foods back in if I know they are going to make me feel terrible?"

I have experimented over the years with adding foods back. For example, I can have spinach and other foods that I had severe, moderate, or minimal reactions to without any issues at all, but gluten is still a no-go for me. If I think to myself, *maybe I am over this gluten sensitivity and I add it into my diet*, joint pain ensues.

But the wealth of knowledge that Kelly and I have gained from our experiences helps guide us on a daily basis, so we can make the choices that will help us feel the best we can feel in the short and long run. To find out how to order the ALCAT, email info@newyouhealthandwellness.com.

Nutrient Deficiencies, Supplements, and Pain

In recent months, along with the ALCAT, I have also suggested that some of my patients undergo micronutrient testing to help them determine what they may be lacking in their diet or supplementation program that could either be contributing to pain or could help decrease their pain.

Here's several examples of some of those nutrients:

VITAMIN D DEFICIENCY

- Role: Vitamin D is crucial for bone health because it helps in the absorption of calcium.
- Impact: A deficiency can lead to osteomalacia in adults, which causes bone pain and muscle weakness. It can also contribute to osteoporosis, increasing the risk of fractures and joint pain.

CALCIUM DEFICIENCY

- Role: Calcium is essential for maintaining strong bones.
- Impact: Inadequate calcium intake can lead to decreased bone density (osteopenia) and osteoporosis, resulting in joint pain and increased susceptibility to fractures/broken bones.

VITAMIN C DEFICIENCY

- Role: Vitamin C is necessary for collagen synthesis, which is a vital component of cartilage.
- Impact: Severe deficiency can lead to scurvy, and mild to moderate deficiency may contribute to weakened connective tissue, bleeding gums, and joint pain due to impaired collagen formation.

OMEGA-3 FATTY ACID DEFICIENCY: OMEGA 6 EXCESS

- Role: Omega-3 fatty acids have anti-inflammatory properties.
- Impact: A lack of omega-3s can lead to increased inflammation in the joints, contributing to conditions like arthritis and joint pain.

MAGNESIUM DEFICIENCY

- Role: Magnesium is involved in over 300 biochemical reactions, including those that regulate muscle and nerve function.
- Impact: A deficiency can cause muscle cramps and spasms, which may lead to muscle and joint pain.

IRON DEFICIENCY

- Role: Iron is essential for the production of hemoglobin, which carries oxygen to the body's tissues.
- Impact: Iron deficiency anemia can lead to fatigue and muscle weakness, which can cause joint pain and discomfort.

LACK OF ZINC, SELENIUM, AND CHROMIUM

- Role: helps with conversion of thyroid hormones from T4 to T3.
- Impact: Less than optimal conversion can impact thyroid hormone synthesis, estrogen, testosterone, and progesterone balance, leading to muscle and joint pain.

From the micronutrient testing, either through blood testing or urine, we can see what nutrients may be missing and help our patients find foods to add to their eating plan or personalized supplementation recommendations to meet their unique needs. I do not want my patients to be taking twenty or more supplements a day. (You wouldn't believe the buckets of supplements my patients bring in that were prescribed by other practitioners!) I do my best to **streamline** the supplements based on testing and research.

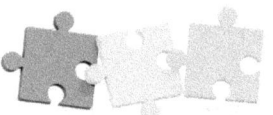

Key Pieces

- **Food Sensitivities and Joint Pain:** Even healthy foods can trigger joint and muscle pain due to food sensitivities, which may cause delayed and varied symptoms, unlike immediate allergic reactions or intolerances.
- **Personalized Reactions:** Each person's microbiome is unique, making their reactions to certain foods different. Food sensitivity testing, like the ALCAT, can help identify specific foods causing inflammation and pain.
- **ALCAT vs. IgG Testing:** The ALCAT is designed to identify food sensitivities by measuring the immune response of white blood cells, providing reliable and actionable results compared to IgG testing, which may only reflect food exposure rather than adverse reactions.
- **Elimination and Healing:** By identifying and removing offending foods, replacing them with nonreactive foods, and reconditioning the gut, patients can significantly reduce joint and muscle pain, improve energy levels, lose weight, and support overall health.

- **Nutrient Deficiencies:** Micronutrient deficiencies, such as vitamin D, omega-3 fatty acids, and magnesium, can exacerbate joint and muscle pain. Addressing these deficiencies through diet and targeted supplementation can improve symptoms.

Want to dig a little deeper?

Go to https://newyouhealthandwellness.com/ebooks/ to find out more about how to use food sensitivity testing to address muscle and joint pain.

CHAPTER 11
How Hormones Cause Joint and Muscle Pain

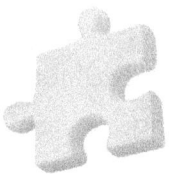

"Hormones get no respect. We think of them as the elusive chemicals that make us a bit moody, but these magical little molecules do so much more."

–Susannah Cahalan

As I sat across from one of my closest friends at a local café, the aroma of freshly brewed coffee wrapped around us. The soft murmur of conversation filled our favorite spot as we drank our soothing hot beverages. Through our conversation, Catherine continued to massage the top of her shoulder, wincing slightly before pausing mid-sentence to fix me with a weary stare.

"I know what you're thinking," she said, a trace of resignation in her voice.

"What? I was listening." I feigned ignorance, as I sipped my chai latte with oat milk.

"Whatever. I know you. You're going to tell me this," she grabbed her upper trapezius muscle, "is my hormones."

I simply shrugged, an unspoken acknowledgment hanging in the air.

"But I told you, the doctor tested my levels. They're fine," she insisted, her voice a mix of frustration and defiance.

"Uh-huh."

"And it's just stress. I have five kids, remember?"

"Yep. I do remember. And I'm running a business, writing a book, and going through a divorce, but I don't have the constant pain you do. I have seen so many patients with that exact issue," I said, as I pointed to her hand, unconsciously massaging the same tight, painful muscles again. I leaned forward, lowering my voice. "The tests they did were just the basics. You need more detailed testing."

She set her cup on the table with a clink, and both palms plopped on the table between us, her expression shifting from irritation to surrender. "Okay, fine. What do you want me to do?"

You've already met Catherine in Chapter 5, when I introduced her hormonal situation that eventually brought us to this discussion in the café. Catherine was finally fed up with her constant muscle pain and general fatigue . . . or maybe she was just fed up with me reminding her about it. The program I had put her on previously helped with the hot flashes and night sweats. That was relatively straightforward, she admitted, so with a bit of prodding she decided to take the next step to get rid of the relentless muscle pain.

Trying to guide friends and family as a practitioner always carries a unique challenge. They see you as their friend, their daughter, or their sibling. They have been there during the times you laughed until you nearly peed your pants. They literally changed your diapers at some point, and well, my mom still sees me as a sixteen-year-old. Many times, they don't see the professional sitting across from them; the one who has supported countless patients over decades.

But Catherine knew more and knew better. She'd been to my clinic as a patient. She had seen my patients on television and knew of the many people we had helped over the years. Yet, resistance wasn't just from her.

Her husband, a physician, was skeptical that someone who was not a medical doctor could possess such nuanced knowledge of hormones, despite the numerous degrees and certificates hanging on my office walls. Moreover, the tests I recommended weren't covered by insurance, meaning any decision carried a financial weight, so for people who rely on insurance only, this can raise red flags in their minds.

As we sat in the warm, comforting buzz of the café, it was clear that this conversation was about more than just skepticism—it was about trust, expertise, and the journey to understanding one's body beyond what conventional wisdom could dictate.

Hormones and Their Effect on Joint and Muscle Health

Most people don't associate hormone issues with joint or muscle health. Instead, many people only think of hormones when they are dealing with their menstrual cycles, fertility issues, menopausal problems, or for men, 'performance issues.'

It usually comes as quite a surprise when I discuss how hormones impact joint and muscle pain.

Because most people are prescribed one or two hormones at a time, it's common to believe that they work separately in the body. Or that taking hormones is just like taking supplements. But that couldn't be further from the truth. Hormones have a significant impact on each other *and* they can have an almost immediate impact on the body, depending on the person taking them.

The interrelationship between hormones is rarely discussed. But Figure 11.1 might give you an idea about how one steroid hormone (often referred to as a sex hormone) is related to another.

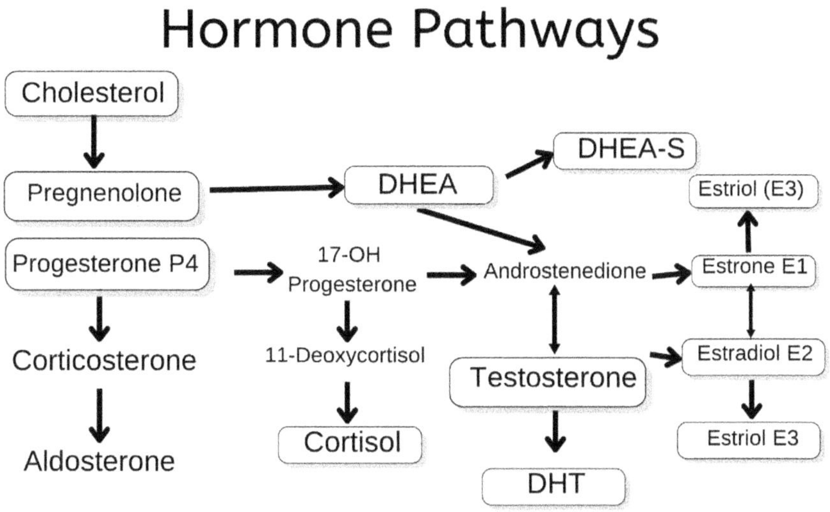

Hormone Pathways

```
Cholesterol
   ↓
Pregnenolone  →  DHEA  →  DHEA-S
   ↓                        Estriol (E3)
Progesterone P4  →  17-OH Progesterone  →  Androstenedione  →  Estrone E1
   ↓                    ↓                        ↑                ↕
Corticosterone    11-Deoxycortisol         Testosterone      Estradiol E2
   ↓                    ↓                        ↓                ↓
Aldosterone         Cortisol                   DHT            Estriol E3
```

Figure 11.1 Steroid hormone pathways. The hormones in boxes are the hormones typically considered when assessing hormone balance.

As you can see, steroid hormone pathways can be quite extensive and complex. And Figure 11.1 is the watered-down version of what these pathways look like. Addressing potential imbalances should be done by taking into consideration what adding one hormone to this cascade can do to other hormones on the pathway. Too often, I see women and men being treated with hormones without taking into consideration how these hormones will impact the hormone above or below them on the diagram in Figure 11.1.

Hormone pathways go beyond even what was shown in the last image. The thyroid and other hormones can be a source of muscle and joint pain, as well.

Thyroid and Muscle Pain

The thyroid is often ignored as a major issue unless completely out of whack and causing a medical emergency, or if you are experiencing fertility issues. The thyroid gland is a major contributor to daily well-being. Its hormones influence everything from your heart rate, body temperature, and metabolism to the production of hormones such as estrogen, progesterone, and testosterone.

If someone has a thyroid diagnosis, it's often called hypothyroid (too little thyroid hormone) or less frequently, hyperthyroid (too much thyroid hormone). And sometimes you hear about autoimmune diseases that affect the thyroid, such as Hashimoto's disease or Graves' disease.

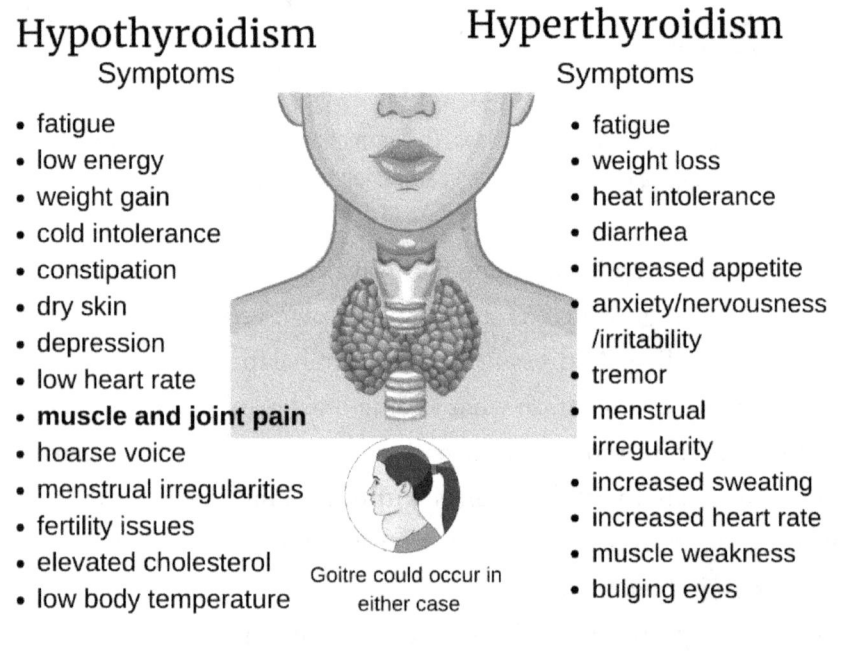

Figure 11.2 Symptoms of hypothyroidism and hyperthyroidism

All of these thyroid-related diagnoses can be related to myalgia, the medical term for muscle pain.

Catherine had constant muscle pain, and as you can tell by the conversation I outlined at the beginning of this chapter, I was convinced it was due to an issue with her thyroid. But despite thyroid blood tests being done, she was told over and over that there was nothing wrong with her thyroid. Many people experience this situation, i.e., you tell your doctor you are tired, sore, gaining weight, your muscles hurt, you feel depressed or anxious, and they do blood tests and tell you that everything is fine.

You're just getting older, they say.

You are going into menopause, they say.

It's a normal part of being a new parent, aging, or _____ (you fill in the blank), they say.

Well, more than a few patients I have seen have told me in one way or another that as they sit with their provider, they may or may not have had a vision of reaching across the table, shutting their provider's laptop or pushing their keyboard and monitor aside, grabbing them and saying, "I am not fine. Please help me!"

But instead, they leave their doctor's office feeling defeated, frustrated, and unsure of what to do next.

When they ask their physician to do detailed testing on the thyroid and not simply the one or two most common blood tests for thyroid function, patients will often get pushback. Occasionally, if the patient presents with many symptoms of thyroid issues and the doctor is sympathetic, trying to appease, or the patient is trying to get pregnant, they may test for free T4. This is the main hormone that the thyroid makes from iodine in the body. It's called T4 due to its four iodine bonds. It is labeled "free" because it has yet to be bound to any other molecules, and if not bound, it is most likely to be absorbed from the blood into the cells and have an impact.

If these two hormone tests come back within normal limits, then regardless of whether the patient has symptom after symptom (see Figure 11.2) commonly related to thyroid issues, no more tests are done, and they are told their thyroid is fine.

That was the exact scenario that Catherine ran into time and time again.

A Shopping Spree

But I had to hand it to her. She finally relented and agreed to get the more extensive tests done. I explained that if her physician continued to refuse to put these blood tests through insurance, the additional tests would require her to pay out-of-pocket. But in her words, she was willing to pay to finally get me to stop bugging her about it. Plus, we made a little wager about what the test results would show.

Due to her consistent and annoying muscle pain, a history of frozen shoulder, a history of endometriosis, her family history of mental health issues, and estrogen-dependent cancer, plus her recent history of hot flashes and significant menopausal symptoms, I was sure the test results would reveal something more about her thyroid. So, before I knew she was ready to do the additional testing, I tried to appeal to her love of shopping and proposed a shopping trip for whoever was right.

"Okay, how about we have a little wager. A new outfit goes to the person who is right. If nothing is wrong with the thyroid, you get a new outfit, my treat. If they find something, you take me shopping and I get the new outfit."

Not something I typically promise to my patients, but between friends, what's wrong with a little incentive?

Catherine later admitted that the new outfit was not the only catalyst for her decision to get some new testing. She reported that she had started doing her own research, and what I was telling her for a year was discussed by other medical professionals, as well.

"You aren't the only crazy person out there," she quipped.

"Yeah, you're funny," I said with a wry smile, while I scribbled on the napkin at the café. "I know I gave these to you before, so just in case you can't find them, here you go." I slid the napkin toward her.

Catherine grabbed the napkin off the table and took my list of the remaining tests to ask her doctor about and put it in her purse.

Catherine took her napkin to the local Any Lab Test Now company, and had the tests that included:

- Thyroid stimulating hormone (TSH) (this previous test was normal)
- Free T4 (FT4)
- Free T3 (FT3)
- Thyroid peroxidase antibodies (TPO)
- Anti-thyroglobulin antibodies (TgAb)

After a couple of days, the results were in.

Her TSH, as before, was normal. Her FT4 levels were normal, but on the low side. Her FT3 levels were normal, but also on the low side. But her thyroid antibodies were elevated. This indicated that, indeed, there was a problem related to her thyroid. Her body was creating antibodies that were attacking her thyroid, and the likelihood that this would eventually lead to hypothyroidism is common. In addition, elevated TPO and TgAb antibodies are correlated with the same muscle pain that Catherine was experiencing.

The Treatment or Lack Thereof

When Catherine took this information back to her primary care doctor, he told her it did not matter. If the TSH wasn't elevated, they wouldn't treat the thyroid medically. When she asked what she should do next, her physician replied that there wasn't anything to do. But once her TSH did become elevated, because her thyroid was failing or had already failed, they would go ahead and start a treatment. So much for an ounce of prevention!

The first time I heard a patient tell me this, I balked at it. I was sure they heard their doctor wrong. But I have heard the same thing repeated by other patients in the exact same scenario who had different physicians in different states, as well as different countries, repeat that same advice. It's not common medical practice to attempt to prevent Hashimoto's disease, the autoimmune issue related to elevated TPO and TgAb, but instead, some physicians will wait until the thyroid fails to function normally as evidenced by elevated TSH levels, and then they will do further testing and consider starting treatment.

Unfortunately, this is an all-too-common conversation my patients have had with their physicians when their thyroid antibodies have been elevated, but not their TSH. I try to educate them about this prior to them seeing their physician as, like me, most of my patients don't believe this is the stance that their doctors will take. It would only be common sense to try to stop a disease process from progressing and prevent the thyroid from failing, right? I wish that were the case.

In Catherine's case, we discussed her options. We started where many are often reluctant to start. We looked at her eating plan.

She had already done a great job of eliminating a lot of the sugary drinks and snacks she had previously been having. This, in addition to adding herbs called adaptogens such as ashwagandha and rehmannia, had significantly improved the hot flashes she was experiencing.

Research has shown that gluten can often be associated with Hashimoto's disease in some people, and eliminating gluten has been shown to significantly improve symptoms related to the disease, and even naturally increase vitamins such as Vitamin D.

Catherine was less than enthused but determined to feel better.

"So, no bread or pasta?"

"Well, you can have some breads and pastas, they just have to be gluten-free."

She bit her lip.

"But you want to make sure they are not processed. Gluten-free packaged food can be full of sugar, additives, and other unhealthy ingredients. Gluten-free doesn't always mean healthy."

A large sigh left Catherine's body.

"Are you sure this is going to work?" she asked. "I have already changed so much," she mumbled, as she sunk back into her seat, her arms folded over her chest.

"I have seen antibodies drop significantly for people following this recommendation. Some have even seen decreases from the thousands back to normal levels. This meant they could have possibly avoided developing a full-blown autoimmune issue."

"It just seems like a lot, especially if we don't know if gluten is really an issue."

Catherine had five kids, and time was always of the essence. I knew she was imagining reading every label of everything she bought on her grocery list for the family. It already took considerable time and energy to prepare large amounts of food for her big crew, and she knew these dishes were often laden with gluten-containing flours, from pastas to breads to bakes. She would have to start changing everything.

"We can do a food sensitivity test first to see if removing gluten is recommended based on those results."

"No, that's okay. That's just more money. I'm just going to have to get used to this."

"That's the spirit," I said, as I leaned over and tapped the desk. Her arms remained folded across her chest. "It will take a couple of months to scope out the substitutes and figure out which gluten-free products you and the kids like."

She was sure of one thing: this was going to be a change for her family. She did not have enough time to make completely separate meals for her kids, herself, and her husband.

"It will probably be good for them, too," she interjected. "The boys are forever farting, and one of the girls has skin issues we can't figure out. With what I read about gluten, this will probably help that too, right?"

"If you have a sensitivity, your kids may be sensitive, as well. But the research is conflicting. If they have a sensitivity or intolerance to gluten, then yes, it could help. It's also important that when gluten is removed, you minimize processed gluten-free foods. After all, most vegetables, salad, and fruits are gluten-free. Therefore, making sure your eating plan is abundant in those foods is important."

"My kids are going to love you," she smirked.

"You may want to consider a probiotic. This is part of our gut reconditioning program."

"I am already on the probiotic, and I would say I do notice feeling lighter around the mid-section, too."

"Great! Then let's get you started with the rest of the program, and we can add in some additional nutrients such as selenium and inositol. These two nutrients together have been shown to be correlated with lower levels of thyroid antibodies." I paused and then continued. "Next time we talk, we can set up the date for my shopping spree."

I felt a smile spread from ear to ear across my face as Catherine appeared to ignore that last comment.

Results . . .

Catherine returned after three months on our program, and two months strictly gluten-free.

She had also gone back for updated thyroid antibody testing.

The test results were sent to me ahead of our appointment, and as she arrived, we sat down to discuss the results.

"How are you feeling?"

Catherine looked at me almost out of the corner of her eye, tilting her head slightly, but she stayed silent.

"Well?" I persisted.

She threw her arms in the air. "Well, I hate to admit it, but I do feel better," she finally replied.

All I could do was smile. Across from me, Catherine crossed her legs, her foot bouncing rhythmically with barely contained energy and a reluctant grin spread across her face. She grabbed her upper trapezius muscles. "And honestly, the muscle pain is essentially gone. I mean, I can still feel that they are tight, but they don't ache anymore."

"Nice!" I exclaimed, as my fingers flew across the keyboard. "Let's review what you have been doing and then we will go over the test results."

Catherine's elevated thyroid antibodies had retreated by 60 percent. Everything was moving in the right direction.

My friend's situation continued to improve over time, with the antibodies coming down to the normal range. Another doctor she found did end up putting her on a low dose of thyroid hormone to help, but the results were headed in the right direction even before the hormone was added.

This isn't as easy a solution for everyone. What if your doctor ordered the thyroid tests, and everything came back within normal limits, including the antibodies? Keep in mind, the thyroid isn't the only gland associated with joint or muscle pain.

Sex Hormones: Menopause, the Menstrual Cycle, and Andropause, Oh My!

As Leslie sat in the chair opposite me, her fingers tapped lightly on the armrests while she surveyed the sea breeze–colored walls of my office. The soft hue, reminiscent of tranquil coastal waters, seemed at odds with the frustration etched on her face. Her eyes darted to the wall lined with windows, briefly catching a glimpse of the outside world before returning to me, seated behind my desk.

"Hi Leslie, it's good to see you. But I am so sorry it's under these circumstances," I said, as I rolled my chair closer to my desk.

She shifted in her seat, wincing slightly as she adjusted her position. "Yeah, me too. I'm back because my left shoulder and elbow are starting to hurt now, and I remember you mentioning something about some of my pain being related to me stopping the pill a couple of months ago. I had been on it forever," she reminded me, her voice tinged with exasperation. ""After I had the SoftWave treatments to my elbow everything seemed fine, at first. I mean, I could still feel it, I could still feel it, but it was close to nothing, and I was able to play pickleball. But recently, my left elbow started hurting, and as you know, I am right-handed, so it clearly wasn't pickleball."

I nodded, leaning forward. "Tell me more about the pain in your left elbow and shoulder, was there an injury; a fall or . . .?" I prompted gently.

"No injury. It just hurts like the right elbow did. And now the shoulder. This just sucks." She sighed, resting her left hand on her right shoulder while supporting her left elbow with her right hand as she spoke. "It's a constant ache that gets worse with movement. It's so frustrating! As soon as I think I'm getting better, something else pops up."

Leslie's eyes conveyed a mix of confusion and irritation. "It's like my body is playing a cruel trick on me, shifting the pain from one spot to another just to tick me off."

She paused and took a deep breath, let it out and continued. "I just want to understand why this is happening. Does it have to do with stopping the pill? And why does it feel like it's just one thing after another?"

As Leslie recounted her experience, it was as if I could see the invisible thread of pain weaving through her life, tugging at different parts of her body, leaving her feeling vulnerable and uncertain. Her story was not just about physical pain, but also about the emotional toll it had taken on her well-being.

Perimenopause and Menopausal Musculoskeletal Pain

I ask women who come to see me what they think is the most common symptom that females experience during menopause. Across the board, the answer is usually hot flashes. There are hundreds of remedies, including hormone replacement, that are constantly making headlines across the airwaves every hour of every day talking about hot flashes related to menopause. But a painful little secret about menopause is musculoskeletal pain, i.e., pain in the muscles and joints can be even more prominent in perimenopause and menopause than hot flashes. In a study that looked at over 300 women with and without diabetes, 78 percent of the women who did not have diabetes reported muscle and joint pain, and 76 percent reported hot flashes.

Another study about menopausal women from 2020 reviewed results from nearly 6,000 participants and revealed that musculoskeletal pain was reported in 71 percent of the women.

So, there you have it: muscle and joint pain is prevalent in women experiencing both perimenopause and menopause. But why?

Sex Hormones are Not Just for Sex

While women have their menstrual cycle, complaints abound about having a period. Society and subsequently our relatives and peers often equate having a menstrual cycle to, at a minimum, an inconvenience, or at its worst, a debilitating pain that steals a week of your life (or more) each month. We take pills, inject pellets, or get shots to oftentimes avoid menstruation. It's the constant nagging 'friend' that visits once a month to make some of our lives miserable. Women tend to look forward to the time our cycle ends. Because at that time, things must get better . . . right? I mean, how bad could hot flashes and some vaginal dryness or pelvic pain really be?

But then it happens, and for the 50 to 70 percent of women who have symptoms in menopause, some start to think that maybe that monthly inconvenience we had when we were younger, for some, wasn't that bad after all.

Estrogen: The Female Hormone

I'll get into the other hormones in more detail, but I am going to start with estrogen. We often think of this hormone as only related to development of breasts, creating eggs, and its fluctuations impacting our menstrual cycle. You may have learned in school that during the early development of a fetus, the gonads (ovaries for females and testicles for males) don't express sex hormones until the tenth or eleventh week of gestation. The expression of these hormones leads to the development of either female or male genitalia. Then, as the baby gets closer to birth and genitalia is developed, the levels of hormones drop off until both estrogen and testosterone come bursting onto the scene in puberty allowing for further differentiation into male and female characteristics.

Estrogen in women, though produced mostly from the ovaries and to a lesser extent by the adrenal glands, doesn't come on the scene on its own. It's converted into estrogen from testosterone, which is also influenced by progesterone. There is a symbiotic relationship between all of these hormones. Men have estrogen too, albeit at much lower levels. See Figure 11.3 for a reminder about the hormone pathway.

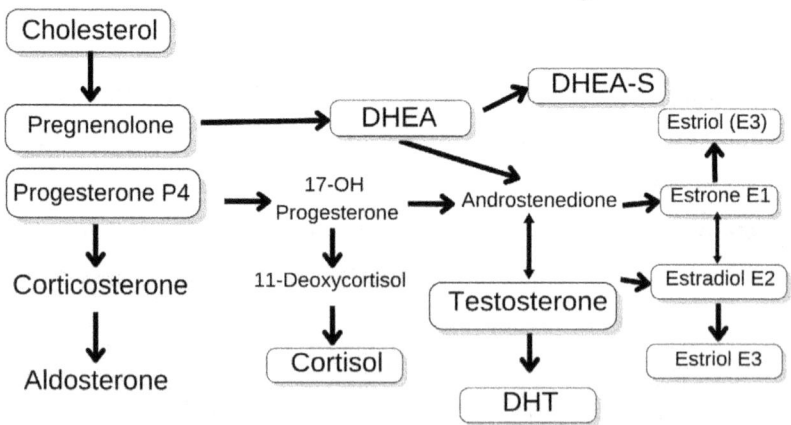

Figure 11.3 Steroid Hormone Pathway: The hormones derived from cholesterol are referred to as steroid hormones or sex hormones.

Estrogen is produced in women during childbearing years mostly from the ovaries and developing eggs. Despite being partly responsible for subsequent ovulation (the brain has to initiate the release of hormones to influence menstruation), estrogen is also responsible for many qualities females often appreciate only when we start losing their effects in menopause.

Estrogen in women helps:

- With bone development
- Support cardiovascular health
- Keep the skin and tissues supple and elastic
- Optimize brain health
- Protect against low-grade inflammation
- Regulate glucose levels
- And more…

You can see that as estrogen decreases, we can end up with increased risk of bone loss (osteoporosis), heart issues, skin changes, brain fog, weight gain, and increased inflammation that can be both local and systemic.

When women enter perimenopause and advance to menopause, the phrase, "You don't know what you got 'til it's gone" certainly rings true. We don't appreciate it when we have it, and we don't (and aren't taught to) support the transition to menopause by making changes earlier to help with the shift our body will be going through. But don't lose hope! Thankfully, changes implemented now, no matter how far into menopause or post-menopause you are, can absolutely improve your situation.

Sex Hormones' Far Reaching Effects

Leslie did not have any indications that she needed a hysterectomy or removal of her ovaries. So, for her, the biggest issue when she saw me was the increased frequency of pain in muscles and joints during perimenopause. As already discussed, this is a common complaint that over 70 percent of women can have during perimenopause (the period of time in your forties when cycles become irregular), menopause (the twelve months where the period stops and doesn't return), and post menopause (the months and years after that twelve months without a cycle). Pain can manifest in muscles, joints, and bones, significantly impacting quality of life.

One of the primary reasons for this increased pain is the fluctuation and decline in hormone levels, particularly estrogen, progesterone, and testosterone. All of these hormones play crucial roles in regulating pain and inflammation. Estrogen, for example, helps to reduce inflammation and maintains joint and muscle health by lubricating joints and supporting muscle mass. As estrogen levels drop during menopause, women can experience increased inflammation and joint stiffness, leading to pain.

Progesterone has an anti-inflammatory effect and a relaxation effect, as well. Lowering levels of progesterone can contribute to increased inflammation, increased swelling in joints, general water retention, and increased muscle tension. And in an analysis of over 10,000 people, low testosterone levels were associated with increased likelihood of having arthritis.

Patients like Leslie tell me that this pain often fluctuates from one area to the next, comes out of nowhere, or seems to be higher than what it should be or has been in the past.

Additionally, the loss of estrogen and progesterone can be related to decreased muscle mass, decrease in ligament tensile strength (ligaments can be torn more easily), and decreased bone density. Women can lose 10 to 20 percent of their lean body mass during perimenopause (the timeframe leading up to menopause when both progesterone and estrogen begin to lower). This loss of muscle mass can cause muscle weakness and joint instability, increasing the risk of injury with activity and exacerbating pain.

The reduction in bone density also raises the risk of osteoporosis, which can cause painful fractures and contribute to chronic pain conditions.

Another factor is the potential development or worsening of conditions such as osteoarthritis and fibromyalgia during this transitional phase. Osteoarthritis (OA) is often thought of as the wear and tear of cartilage in joints, but evidence is showing that well-worn explanation may be approaching its use-by date. OA seems to be more prevalent in postmenopausal women due to the protective effects of estrogen being diminished. And we have already discussed in Chapter 9 the impact of increased LPS on systemic and localized inflammation in the body, but estrogen is protective against the damage of LPS. Therefore, as our estrogen levels fall, a protection against degeneration from LPS decreases too, leaving us more susceptible to joint and muscle pain.

While discussing gut health in Chapter 9, you also learned that the changes in estrogen levels affect the microbiome and contribute to the changes in the gut-joint axis. This also can contribute to or worsen the degeneration of joint cartilage, causing pain.

Hormone Imbalance and Pain

Do you remember Steve? You met him at the beginning of this book. He hurt his back bending over and had issues with continued pain, eventually coming off medications like opioids that were making him constipated and lethargic. He also noticed increased sensitivity to pain in general while trying to get off the opioids, meaning he was experiencing hypersensitivity to pain overall. This scared him.

While Leslie was not overweight, after checking her estrogen and progesterone levels, her estrogen was nearly undetectable, and progesterone was extremely low. Her testosterone was on the low side of normal. Thyroid tests (all of them), adrenal testing (cortisol and DHEA), and her HbA1c (a measure of her average blood sugar over the last three months) came back normal, even optimal. The feedback inhibition that was caused by long-term oral contraceptive use resulted in her estrogen and progesterone levels being extremely low. Many times, other organ systems are involved, but in Leslie's case her other systems seemed to be running along fine.

> Feedback inhibition is a natural process in the body. It is one of the ways hormones are kept in balance. It will come into play again later in this chapter when I discuss whether taking hormones is the best choice to rid yourself of muscle and joint pain.
>
> But for now, think of feedback inhibition or negative feedback as a mechanism that helps keep balance in the body. If one hormone is low in the blood, the brain senses this and signals to the responsible organ system to make more of the hormone that is needed.
>
> When the hormone gets to the point where there is enough of it in the bloodstream, the brain slows down the production of its signaling hormone.
>
> This is the body's innate balancing act.

Steve, on the other hand, was overweight. When he had checked his free testosterone levels, they were quite low. This often occurs in overweight or obese men and men who have been under stress for long periods of time. I asked him to go back to the doctor to also check his estrogen levels because in men, low testosterone can result from increased activity of an enzyme called the aromatase. In men, this can result in testosterone converting into too much estrogen, which is not good for men. Higher than normal estrogen in men can result in:

- Weight gain
- Enlarged prostate
- Breast development
- Muscle atrophy

- Decreased libido
- Sexual dysfunction
- Fatigue
- Brain fog
- Hair loss
- Mood swings
- Joint pain
- And more...

His blood tests showed low total and free testosterone, high estradiol, and low DHEA (testosterone comes from DHEA). His thyroid and cortisol levels were normal, but on the low side.

The Solution

Both of these patients underwent an overview of their eating plans. Steve did the ALCAT food sensitivity test, and we looked at his micronutrient levels. He was significantly low in zinc and Vitamin D. These nutrients are essential for maintaining testosterone levels in men. I suggested he take a good quality multivitamin with these nutrients including magnesium, as that has been shown to support the levels of testosterone in men, as well. We added a probiotic and our gut reconditioning program to improve his overall gut health since he had been on opioids, which tend to cause constipation. We also added a fish oil supplement to help with inflammation.

Because Steve's estrogen levels were elevated for a male, and since this can be related to inflammation, potential prostate issues, and other symptoms, we put Steve on a supplement called diindolylmethane (DIM), the active ingredient in cruciferous vegetables. He hadn't shown any sensitivity to these vegetables, and DIM can assist in slowing down the conversion of testosterone to estrogen. Many times, this ends up improving testosterone levels and normalizing estrogen levels in men. One word of caution: I have had patients who were taking other medications for other health issues, and if these medications impact the liver, then DIM may cause them to feel unwell. Therefore, make sure you check with your healthcare provider before starting with this or any other supplement.

Because SoftWave, our electrohydraulic shockwave device, did not help Steve significantly after three or four treatments, we shifted to looking at his eating plan. After three months of sticking to his ALCAT information, adjusting his eating plan, and taking the supplementation, Steve finally felt like he was coming out of his slump. His sleep improved, weight started to come off, and he started to exercise again because his back was consistently feeling better. We caught up six months after starting the new eating plan, supplements, and exercise, and he reported occasional back pain that he was able to manage by doing his exercises and avoiding the foods that he now knew caused the pain to flare up. At this point, he was keen to begin SoftWave again to see if it helped now that the overall inflammation in his body was down and the pain was significantly less and intermittent. We were both pleasantly surprised when he was pain-free after an additional three SoftWave treatments, combined with advancing his abdominal stabilization program. Prior to this, he had not reacted well to SoftWave and any abdominal stabilization exercise increased his symptoms. Thankfully, that was no longer the case.

For Leslie, she did not feel her eating plan was a big issue, so she decided to wait on doing the food sensitivity or micronutrient testing. She had been eating a healthy Mediterranean diet and decided to continue that and eliminate alcohol consumption for three months. She stopped having her daily sugary treats and limited herself to dark chocolate once or twice a week. She also did our cleanse during this time to improve her gut health.

After her estrogen and progesterone levels showed they were extremely low, we had a discussion about whether hormone therapy was an option for her. She chose to adjust her diet and took herbals called shatavari and chaste tree berry to assist with her estrogen and progesterone since she wanted to give her body a break from taking hormones. She understood these herbs were not going to move her hormone levels to what they were prior to taking the pill, but she wanted to try them first before considering hormone replacement. Leslie was already taking a good quality fish oil supplement, a reputable multivitamin, and a potent probiotic. We continued to do SoftWave, the electrohydraulic shockwave device, and she responded very well again to the treatment.

She opted to join our membership program where she would receive one SoftWave treatment per month, and at her six-month follow-up, she wasn't sure what to treat as both her elbows and her shoulder were feeling good.

After a few months, Leslie was able to stop wearing her elbow brace on her right side while she played pickleball, and she was still off alcohol because she noticed that she felt achy in general after having it. This was the last month that we reviewed her eating plan to balance her proteins, low glycemic carbohydrates, and good fats, and she stayed consistent with her supplementation program. Leslie opted not to redo her hormone testing because she was feeling well.

We both agreed that her progress was fantastic. I let her know she could continue maintenance for prevention, utilize our other services with a membership or come back in the future if she needed any other treatment.

But I do remind her every time I see her to retest her hormones once every six months or so to keep track of these levels because hormone replacement at some point may be a necessary intervention for her if symptoms returned.

When we did further assessment of Steve's testosterone levels, as his weight gradually came off from exercising more due to being pain free, his testosterone levels increased, and his estrogen levels decreased. He felt like he had a new lease on life as long as he stayed close to his eating plan.

Both Steve and Leslie had been on a strength-training program. Leslie liked to do her program at the gym, and Steve preferred to work out at home. They had come a long way, and by following the system, each had tremendous improvements. It wasn't easy, and like me, they had their struggles and tested their boundaries with eating foods they knew weren't the best for them. They admitted, like I do, that they usually paid for it, as their joints or muscles would remind them that they had crossed the line. But overall, they knew that they had to love the way they felt without those foods and drinks more than they disliked the inconvenience of doing what was necessary to optimize their gut, hormone, and joint health.

Could Hormone Replacement Be the Answer?

The short answer is, potentially, yes. For example, Catherine replaced her thyroid hormone with a low dose of that hormone after her antibodies started to come down. Changing her eating plan, adding relevant supplementation, and adding thyroid hormone brought her antibodies down and helped her to avoid developing Hashimoto's disease.

But if you use hormone replacement before addressing underlying causes of why hormones are an issue in the first place, then hormone replacement becomes a Band-Aid, just like other medications that don't address the true root cause of an issue. Hormone replacement (in some cases) can help you feel better but may just be a temporary fix covering up the real culprit instead of being a long-term solution.

Take Amy, for example. She felt better after our SoftWave treatment of her thumb and neck pain, but the symptoms continued to return. She

HOW HORMONES CAUSE JOINT AND MUSCLE PAIN

had gut issues, including irritable bowel syndrome, but was resistant to address her gut health or her eating plan, even after spending money on the ALCAT test. Amy, unfortunately, never followed through on implementing the changes suggested based on the findings of the ALCAT.

Despite my continued explanation of how her gut health and eating plan could be impacting her situation, she resisted changing anything related to these topics. But Amy was much more interested in the information that I discussed about hormones and how they can contribute to joint pain.

Amy stopped coming to see me for over six months, and one afternoon, she showed up to the clinic with the same neck problem I had treated months earlier.

She happily reported that after we spoke about hormones and the potential issues they can create related to joint pain, she went to a clinic that prescribed hormone therapy for menopausal issues. No testing was done, and she was prescribed estradiol and progesterone based on her symptoms. Her overall joint pain had subsided within a few weeks and some joint pain had gone away completely . . . at first. But six months later, her neck pain in particular was starting to surface again.

Amy hadn't changed her diet or implemented any of the suggestions regarding her eating plan and supplementation. Amy had also not had her hormone levels tested after starting the hormonal treatment six months prior, so I offered her an opportunity to have the tests done through our clinic to see where her levels were sitting now. My concern was that there might be too much hormone building up in her tissues, or too little, if her body had accommodated or basically got used to the dose that she was taking. Keep in mind, she still had not addressed the IBS symptoms with her diet and continued to have this issue.

Despite me suggesting that she address her gut, eating plan, and optimizing her hormone production naturally, she did not want any part of it and just wanted to do SoftWave. We started treatment and once again, unlike more than 80 percent of my patients who get significant long-lasting relief from SoftWave, our manual therapy, and exercise, Amy reported some improvement with her neck pain, but the pain continued to return after just a few hours.

She had one SoftWave treatment left in the package that she purchased and out of sheer frustration (and part of me was convinced she wanted to prove me wrong), Amy started to implement the gut reconditioning program and work on her eating plan.

After three months of implementing these changes, Amy came back for the last visit in her package for SoftWave and manual therapy sessions. To her utter surprise, after the last treatment in her package, the neck pain was now completely gone and had stayed away this time for nearly three weeks.

She decided to do three more treatments since her results were so much better this time around.

Her doctor did not feel it was necessary to retest her hormone levels, so she pursued the urinary testing that we offer. Amy's estrogen levels were in the high normal range, while progesterone sat at the low end of normal. Her testosterone was low normal, as well.

Amy continues to monitor her hormone levels through our clinic every six months and takes these results to her prescribing physician to adjust doses when needed. Her eating plan continues to be a work in progress.

The Advantages of Hormone Replacement

The obvious advantage of utilizing hormones to replace the ones that are low is related to exactly what Amy experienced. Within the first two weeks of taking the hormones estrogen and progesterone (even without doing anything about her eating plan and gut health), Amy felt better. Her perimenopausal symptoms of hot flashes, joint pain, and even her irritable bowel symptoms decreased and some of the symptoms were kept at bay.

Another advantage was that the physician could prescribe hormone therapy without needing blood tests or urine tests to back up reason to prescribe. Experiencing menopausal-like symptoms are sufficient, many times, to receive a prescription. And hormone replacement therapy (HRT) can be covered by insurance.

Research shows that HRT, when prescribed correctly, may be protective against other issues such as cardiovascular disease, osteoporosis, and type 2 diabetes.

If low hormones are the cause of anxiety or depression, HRT may help with those diagnosis as well, and there are some studies showing it can improve sleep.

And thankfully, according to Dr. Lisa Mosconi, author of *The Menopause Brain*, "There is little evidence that the combination of bioidentical estrogen and progesterone increases the risk of breast cancer."

Bioidentical refers to hormones made from plant sources that have the same chemical structure as those hormones found in our own bodies.

The Disadvantages of Hormone Replacement

Let's use Amy's experience first.

First and foremost, if the true underlying cause of symptoms aren't addressed first, HRT can act like a Band-Aid, covering up symptoms for a while, only to have them return months or a year or so later.

For Amy, her bowel symptoms and her joint pain returned, especially the nagging discomfort in her neck that kept her from having a good night's sleep.

Why would her symptoms return? Because the hormones in perimenopause weren't the true underlying cause of all of her symptoms.

Some would challenge me and say that perimenopause and even menopause are the underlying cause of the low hormones. 'They' may say that if a woman is low in estrogen or progesterone because of perimenopause or menopause, giving them those hormones is addressing the cause.

However, 25 to 40 percent of women go through menopause without issue, so can we really say the lowering of these hormones in menopause is the main or root cause of all their symptoms? Or are some menopausal symptoms just an effect of other factors that, if addressed, would naturally improve the balance of the hormones the body is still producing in menopause and alleviate symptoms? After all, if not everyone experiences joint pain, hot flashes, or other menopausal issues, but every woman's estrogen and progesterone levels lower in menopause, then what is the reason that some women experience the symptoms and others do not? Genetics? Maybe, but I'm not convinced that is the entire story, especially when I see these symptoms disappear after adjusting the eating plan, addressing stress, and optimizing gut health.

Shouldn't these lifestyle changes be the first line of defense against the symptoms of perimenopause and menopause?

But you might say, what's the big deal? If hormones address the symptoms and they don't have serious side effects, then no harm, no foul, right?

Well, not exactly.

The Seldom-Discussed Disadvantage of Any Hormone Replacement: Feedback Inhibition

Stan arrived at the clinic as he did every month for his erectile dysfunction (ED) treatment maintenance session. He was in his early forties and was experiencing pelvic pain and what he thought was ED, but it turned out to be more of a pelvic floor dysfunction.

Our true shockwave device treatment, plus pelvic health physical therapy, was the ticket to helping him be pain-free and improve his performance. He chose to continue with monthly treatments to maintain his progress and keep himself accountable to doing his exercises and lifestyle changes.

But on one day in particular, Stan did not seem like himself. He was fidgeting a bit and seemed uncomfortable. We had built a good rapport, and this was in stark contrast to what our normal appointments were like.

"How are you doing Stan?" I asked.

"I am okay, good, I guess," he replied.

"Are you sure everything is okay? You seem a little... uncomfortable?"

After hemming and hawing a little bit, he finally spoke up. "This is really kind of difficult for me to talk about. And I am a little freaked out."

"Well, okay. You don't have to talk to me about it if it makes you uncomfortable, but just know that I am here to listen."

"I actually need to talk to you about it." He paused, and his chest rose slowly and fell quickly. He avoided eye contact with me and continued, "Because it has to do with my, umm, testicles."

"Are you experiencing pelvic pain like you had previously?" I asked.

"No, that's not it." His brow wrinkled, and his eyes opened a little wider. "Remember a while back, I told you I was considering taking testosterone to help with libido."

"Yes."

"I did not tell you last time because I wasn't sure if you would think it's a good idea. But the doctor put me on some pellets, and I looked it up and the dosage is pretty high."

"Okay," I reassured him. "I am not against hormone therapy, so I am glad you told me. But you said your testicles were an issue. Can you tell me what the problem is?"

I had an idea but wanted to give Stan the opportunity to share his concern.

"They don't hurt at all. It's just that," he cleared his throat and met my eyes. "They have basically shrunk."

I stopped typing on my laptop. "That is quite common, Stan," I replied.

"You see, when you take a hormone like testosterone, or any hormone for that matter, your body gradually decreases the amount of that hormone that you normally make. It's called feedback inhibition. Since the body is getting a regular dose of testosterone from your pellets, the brain is receiving a message that you have plenty of testosterone. The brain then either slows down or stops sending a signal to your testicles, since that is the where testosterone is produced. The result is that you make significantly less hormone, and this can wind up causing the testicles to shrink. The factory down there basically goes on an extended vacation, and in many men, sperm production slows or stops completely."

Stan's shoulders fell and he leaned forward, resting his forearms on my desk. He lowered his voice slightly and asked, "Will my testicles stay this way?"

"Research suggests that stopping short-term testosterone use results in return of sperm production in men within six to twenty-four months. But the longer a man is on testosterone therapy and the older he is, the less likely his fertility is to return to normal. Once the testosterone therapy is stopped and the testicles resume their own production, if possible, they should return back to normal size," I explained.

Feedback inhibition doesn't only affect men taking testosterone, it can potentially impact anyone taking hormones.

In women, oral contraceptive pills (OCP) result in feedback inhibition. This is one reason why a woman on birth control doesn't typically release a viable egg or produce a healthy enough lining to sustain a pregnancy. Her own hormone production is slowed significantly when taking oral contraception, as these pills contain estrogen, progesterone, or a combination of both.

Taking hormones orally, receiving injections or pellets, or using an IUD such as the Mirena (that releases a synthetic hormone called progestin) results in the suppression of hormones from the brain that typically signal estrogen and progesterone production.

For many women, when they come off OCP, the feedback inhibition is reversed, and they usually start their cycle again within twelve months. But for some it can take much longer.

However, prolonged use of contraception—whether due to starting at a younger age, using the pill to skip periods, or continuing oral contraceptives after completing their family—can lead to additional side effects.

These include, but are not limited to:

- Low libido
- Vaginal atrophy (atrophic vaginitis) and thinning of the vaginal tissue
- Thinning labia

Using hormone creams such as estrogen on the vaginal tissue can address the vaginal atrophy, and thankfully research has shown it is not related to an increased risk of breast cancer, as previously thought.

But hormone creams or oral intake of hormones can affect the entire body systemically. So, though women may find relief from hot flashes, vaginal symptoms, and perhaps joint pain with hormone replacement, if the underlying cause of these problems is not addressed, symptoms will likely come back at some point. But the fact that the symptoms return while on the hormone replacement again supports the premise that the underlying issue causing these symptoms is not being fully addressed.

Feedback inhibition may contribute to additional hormone issues, and without proper monitoring of hormones prior to and during HRT, staying on the hormones could lead to lower production of hormones naturally and result in making it difficult to come off the hormones without symptoms returning.

The latter can also be a sign that the true underlying causes of the symptoms are not being addressed. Appropriate monitoring of hormone levels may help to avoid the return of menopausal symptoms including joint pain. But monitoring could also prevent creating another hormone imbalance, either by overuse or the hormones converting into another hormone instead of being available for the hormone that was low in the first place.

The Importance of Monitoring HRT

Sylvia was a perimenopausal forty-something and showed up in my office an absolute wreck. She was a longtime patient, and I had never seen her in this condition. I can't even put our conversation into words because it was so erratic. Even on that day, it wasn't making a lot of sense to me.

When Sylvia arrived very distraught, her eyes were red and puffy, and she looked exhausted. After I cautiously asked her how she was, she immediately began to cry.

When I asked her what was going on, she could barely string a sentence together.

I knew Sylvia had been using progesterone cream for the previous six months to help with her perimenopausal symptoms. I had been seeing her for her knee and shoulder previously, and she was responding extremely well to SoftWave treatment, manual therapy, and exercise. But on that day, I wasn't sure how we were going to get through the treatment.

After using up half the session to decipher what was happening to Sylvia emotionally, I finally pieced together that she and her long-term boyfriend had recently broken up. But even with that happening, I had a feeling this response was not consistent with her demeanor when she had been upset in the past. I asked her if she was still taking the progesterone cream, and whether they had monitored how it was affecting her system via urine tests or saliva testing.

She shook her head. I suggested she have her hormones tested as soon as she felt up to it, and since her knee was doing so well, to take some time to deal with the recent breakup. Four weeks later she returned to the clinic looking better and was able to hold a normal conversation. She confessed that when she started taking the progesterone cream, she noticed that she was feeling better, so she increased the dose on her own. "Just slightly," she said.

But when Sylvia gave me her test results, her progesterone levels had been ten times what they should be. This would explain the aberrant behavior I had witnessed the last time I saw her. When she took progesterone and increased it prematurely, not only did she experience feedback inhibition, but it appeared that the hormone may have been building up in her tissues. Steroid hormones, like progesterone, are fat soluble, so they can have the tendency to rise in the system if too much is being taken or if a significant amount is being made internally and the body is unable to clear them efficiently.

Sylvia revealed that once she received the test results and saw the high levels, she stopped the cream and recently started using it again, albeit at a much lower dose. She slowly started to feel back to normal. "I still cry because of the breakup, but it's not uncontrollable like it was."

Hormone replacement therapy should be monitored closely. If taken by injection, through pellets, or from patches, serum blood tests can be a good way to obtain a baseline, but there is some evidence that if taken orally or with creams, urine testing can have some advantages.

When I see patients to help them optimize hormone balance, we use a combination of blood and urine tests. Blood tests are often just a snapshot of what a hormone is doing at a particular time, while urine and saliva tests can be done throughout the day to assess the patient's hormone fluctuation, which turns out is a helpful bit of information. For example, Sylvia's blood results showed her progesterone levels were on the high side of normal but not out of the 'normal' range, but her urine testing showed significantly high progesterone levels and high progesterone metabolites. Metabolites are the substances hormones break down into when they are being cleared by the body.

I run into too many people that take hormones for months and even years without follow-up testing. This is not a responsible practice in my opinion. Hormones like testosterone, progesterone, and estrogen are not like many supplements that are excreted from the body easily. Their breakdown and elimination or reuse by the body is a more complex and slower process.

Another Issue When There Is Improper Hormone Monitoring

Another issue related to hormone replacement therapy is not necessarily the hormones themselves, but the knowledge of the person prescribing them.

It is common knowledge that physicians who treat women who have had estrogen-dependent cancers, such as breast cancer, are extremely cautious and often recommend against hormone replacement therapy, especially those that contain estrogen. This is a prudent caution and the decision of whether to take any hormone replacement in these cases should be discussed with the prescribing physician and the oncologist.

Where I typically see a problem with prescribing hormones, besides not addressing the true underlying cause of hormone depletion first, is when men or women are prescribed hormone therapies without the prescriber taking into account how one hormone impacts another.

For example, as you saw earlier in the images of the hormone cascade in Figures 11.1 and 11.3, cholesterol converts into other hormones including progesterone, estrogen, and testosterone. But what I see happening too often is if a blood test shows that one of these three hormones is low, the person will be prescribed that hormone without taking into consideration how the addition of that hormone may affect the ones above or below it in the chain.

Let's look at the hormone pathway again.

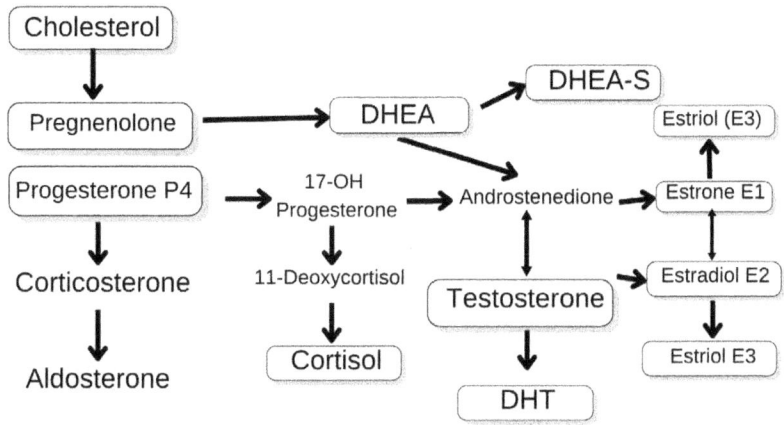

Figure 11.3 Steroid Hormone Pathway

Are you tired of seeing this image yet? It's important to always keep in mind how hormones affect each other.

In clinic, I see testosterone prescribed when it's low, even if estrogen is normal or high. But if testosterone is low and we haven't addressed why it is low (is it thyroid? is it cortisol, is it converting too quickly to estrogen? is DHEA low? what else can be contributing?), then taking testosterone may just end up converting into more estrogen, creating a bigger problem of too much estrogen in the body.

This can lead to many symptoms and issues such as worsening premenstrual symptoms, breast soreness and cystic breasts, fibroids, endometriosis, irritability, joint and muscle pain, and more.

If a male has low testosterone and he is prescribed testosterone without trying to figure out why it is low and addressing that first, his testosterone could just convert into estradiol and down the line cause prostate issues, breast enlargement, decreased energy, irritability, and more. This is exactly what happened to Stan, who you met earlier. He started taking testosterone and was concerned about his testicles shrinking in size. But besides that issue, he also confided in me that the clinic where he got his pellets was monitoring only his testosterone, not his estrogen. So, when they saw that despite him taking a significant amount of testosterone, his testosterone levels weren't improving to the level they wanted them to be, instead of checking why (i.e., where was the testosterone going?), they just kept increasing the dose.

It turns out that his testosterone was converting into higher levels of two types of estrogen, which, if it was not addressed, may have caused significant health issues. Like Steve, who had low testosterone, we added a supplement called diindolylmethane (DIM). This supplement is made from the active ingredient in cruciferous vegetables like broccoli and cauliflower, and after he began taking it, Stan's estrogen started to decrease, his testosterone increased, and he was able to decrease the dose of testosterone he was getting from the clinic.

Here's another example. When a woman presents with low progesterone due to high cortisol levels (progesterone can be converted into cortisol during times of stress), giving her progesterone may help in the short term, but if she doesn't address the trigger (tangible or intangible), i.e., what is causing the stress, and this trigger continues, the increased catabolic (breaking down) effects of cortisol could contribute to long-term issues such as bone density problems, weight gain, high blood pressure, anxiety, muscle weakness, and more.

The answer, then, is to make sure whoever is prescribing you hormone replacement is taking into consideration why your hormones are low in the first place (menopause isn't always the reason for symptoms common in menopause) and knows what to do to address what they find, either naturally or with HRT.

Low Hormones Aren't Always the Root Cause of Your Symptoms

For women, don't let the diagnosis of perimenopause or menopause be the only reason you take hormones for symptoms. I say this from personal experience; despite my mom having horrible menopausal symptoms, I haven't had any hot flashes, dryness, skin issues, gut issues, or brain fog on my menopausal journey. And any joint pain that I have can be eliminated through diet and gut health. At the time of this writing, the menopausal middle is starting to creep in, so I will keep you posted on the results of my addressing that, but all in all, I have fared well almost a decade into menopause. Our moms are usually a good barometer about how we will handle menopause, unless you take steps to address these hormonal changes differently than your mom did, which thankfully I had the opportunity to gain the knowledge necessary to avoid a rough patch like my mother had.

All too often, when my patients address their eating plan, and, if needed, focus on gut health by tackling food sensitivities, nutritional deficiencies (and take the right supplementation for them), manage stress, and get on the best exercise program for their situation, menopausal symptoms go away or never show up in the first place.

For men, consider the same. Testosterone isn't always low just because you are forty, fifty, or even sixty-plus years old. The eating plan, nutritional status, stress, and exercise routine could be to blame.

And make sure your provider prescribing the hormones understands how hormones impact each other. That is, make sure they understand how the hormones convert from and into each other and what the upstream or downstream consequences of taking hormones could be in the short or long run. Beware of using hormones as a Band-Aid. Work with someone who will work with you to assess and address the underlying causes.

How Long Do I Have to Stay on Hormone Replacement?

The length of time someone would need to stay on hormone replacement to achieve and maintain the desired results varies. Thyroid hormones, for example, which are yet another type of hormone called tyrosine-based hormones, work together with steroid and peptide hormones to coordinate complex physiological processes in response to many different stimuli, both in and outside of the body.

Someone like me is likely to stay on thyroid hormones for the duration of their lives. With lifestyle changes, I have been able to reduce my dose of thyroid hormone to a lower dose where I feel well and energetic. When I wasn't paying as close attention to food sensitivities and my gut health, for example, my blood tests were showing that I needed more and more thyroid hormone. To avoid that slippery slope now and in the future, I stay committed to the eating plan that best suits my body, not my emotional cravings.

Do I fall off the wagon occasionally? Yes, I am human. But my body quickly reminds me with knee, back, and leg pain, as well as whole-body aches when I stray from what is best. My point here is that some hormones, like thyroid hormones due to feedback inhibition, will likely need to be used for life, unless you can address the issues that potentially caused the thyroid to become off track in the first place early on. Had I known this twenty years ago, I would have made different choices to address my thyroid health naturally first. Then, if that did not work, I would have added thyroid hormone at the smallest amount possible.

For steroid hormones such as estrogen, progesterone, DHEA, and testosterone, these also may require you to be on them for the long term to continue achieving results that you have gotten in the past. However, I have found that if they are taken for the short term while addressing underlying issues causing the very symptoms you are taking the hormones for, it is possible to come off them and feel well. Each person's situation is unique, and any adjustment of hormone dosages should be done with direction from your prescribing physician.

Topical hormones such as estrogen creams or gels to the vagina typically need to be continued to produce the same results over time. But not always. Each person's situation is different. (I know, I say that a lot).

The longer your body depends on a hormone, the harder it can be for some people to come off of them and not feel unwell or have their previous or other symptoms come back. Like women coming off the pill or men coming off testosterone, normal function can take time to come back.

When I attempted to decrease the thyroid hormone that I take, as I got to a very low dose, I noticed my hair began to slowly start falling out. I went back to the previous, yet lower, dose than when I started, the symptoms stabilized, and new hair growth sprouted. I did not have issues with hair falling out before starting thyroid hormone, but that is one of the symptoms related to not enough thyroid hormone in the body.

My patients who stop their hormones on their own, cold turkey, often abruptly crash and feel unwell. Others who wean off the hormones can take weeks or months for symptoms to return, and then feel the effects of stopping their hormone treatment. And others do fine after weaning off completely after a short time on them or find that a much lower dose of the hormone suffices. These women tend to be dedicated to making the changes we discuss in this book.

I always recommend working with a trusted healthcare professional if you want to explore decreasing the hormones you are taking. Never just stop taking them without appropriate testing and assistance to guide you.

What's the Alternative to Hormone Replacement?

The point of this section of *The Pain-Free Formula* was not to tell you to take hormones or not to take them. Instead, I wanted to provide you the information necessary to make an informed decision *before* starting a potentially long-term commitment.

Some of my patients ask me if I am against the use of hormones, and the answer is absolutely not. But what I am against is putting people on hormones as the first line of action without helping them understand what impact this may have on their bodies in the short and long term. Unfortunately, this is rarely done. In my opinion, it is a practitioner's responsibility to counsel patients on what they can do to address the underlying causes, i.e., the tangible and intangible triggers that we have discussed throughout this book, instead of or before using hormones as a treatment.

When to Start HRT as the First Line of Treatment

The one exception to my general rule of addressing the likely root cause of joint pain and other issues related to less-than-optimal hormone production, before starting hormones, is when a patient is just worn down and they do not have the energy or the emotional and physiological resources to make the effort that is needed to start and stick to lifestyle changes. For these patients, starting hormone therapy could be a major plus as they gain the strength to implement changes in their lives.

Many times, these patients can come off the HRT and other times they choose to stay on it. This is a personal decision to be discussed with your trusted healthcare professional. But I caution my patients to avoid using the fact that they feel good in the short term to be an excuse for not addressing their eating plan, gut health, and overall health. Not addressing the underlying issues in this book will likely come back to bite you.

Alternatives to Hormone Replacement

When I discuss feedback inhibition and appropriate monitoring of hormones to assess if the treatment plan is working, patients can get frustrated and ask, "If I don't want to take hormones, what can I do to address hormone issues?"

Thankfully, there are plenty of things that can be done to improve hormone balance without needing to take hormones as the first step.

You have heard me say it before:

- Optimal eating plan (including assessing food sensitivities)
- Optimal supplementation based on your personal needs
- Effective exercise program
- Managing stress (which we cover in the next chapter)

For most, the first place to start is your eating plan. Foods and herbs can be used to address optimal hormone balance. In her book *The Menopause Brain*, Dr. Lisa recommends the Mediterranean diet for its "protective effects on the brain, heart, gut, and hormones."

She also reveals research showing women who ate the traditional standard American diet (SAD) diet with more processed foods and refined carbohydrates like white rice and pasta went into menopause earlier and had more severe symptoms.

There are several supplements that can be utilized as well to address menopausal issues such as chaste tree berry and DIM, which we have already discussed.

Overall, no matter how you decide to tackle your joint pain, the important thing is that you have all the information you need to make the decision that is right for you.

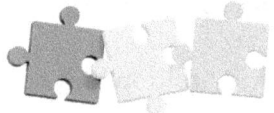

Key Pieces

Hormones and Pain: Hormones like thyroid hormones, estrogen, progesterone, and testosterone play crucial roles in maintaining joint and muscle health. Imbalances or declines in these hormones, especially during perimenopause and menopause, as well as times of stress for both genders can lead to increased inflammation, joint stiffness, and muscle pain.

Feedback Inhibition: Hormone replacement therapy (HRT) can lead to feedback inhibition, where the body reduces its natural hormone production due to the external supply. This can cause long-term reliance on hormone therapy and may lead to other health issues if not properly monitored.

Personalized Treatment: Proper hormone balance involves more than just replacing missing hormones. Addressing underlying causes such as diet, gut health, and stress is crucial for long-term relief from symptoms like joint and muscle pain.

Monitoring HRT: Continuous monitoring of hormone levels is essential when undergoing HRT to obtain a baseline and avoid imbalances and side effects. Hormone therapy should be tailored to the individual, taking into account how one hormone affects others in the body.

Non-Hormonal Alternatives: There are non-hormonal approaches to managing hormone-related joint and muscle pain, including dietary changes, supplementation, exercise, and stress management. These should be considered before or alongside hormone therapy.

Want to dig a little deeper?

Go to https://newyouhealthandwellness.com/ebooks to find out more about how to assess and address your hormones to get rid of muscle and joint pain.

CHAPTER 12

When Stress Takes a Toll
Pain's Hidden Trigger

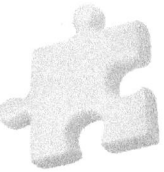

"For fast-acting relief, try slowing down."

–Lily Tomlin

Jennifer, the CEO of a bustling healthcare facility, burst through the front door of our clinic. Her presence was a whirlwind with phone in hand, and an over-the-shoulder briefcase in tow. She had seen our Facebook ad about the SoftWave trial for pain relief, and despite canceling twice before due to work commitments, she was here—albeit late.

From the moment she walked in, her phone seemed like an extension of her hand, constantly buzzing with texts and calls. Apologetically setting it aside with the face down did not stop the interruptions. Her Apple Watch would ping constantly, drawing her attention to her wrist.

"I am so sorry I was late. I was stuck on a Zoom call, then the GPS took me to the wrong address," her voice trailed off, and she slightly lifted her hand from her wrist and glanced down briefly.

With a strained smile, I began to ask her questions about her pain, attempting to hide my frustration behind professional courtesy. Amidst the frequent vibrations buzzing, she finally gently covered her wrist while we talked, and did her best to attempt to ignore the digital tether binding her to work responsibilities.

After a few feeble attempts at a conversation to gain more information, we eventually moved from the desk to the exam table, since I wasn't getting much detailed information due to the constant distractions. As she laid down onto the exam table, I noticed the tension in her posture as she moved rigidly to lie down. But no sooner had she lay supine on the table than she sat up and tapped the Apple watch on her wrist a few times. "Sorry, one sec," she muttered while getting up off the table to grab her phone.

At that point her thumbs began flying across her phone screen before shoving the device into her bag. Jennifer carried her bag back with her and set it onto the side of the exam table and resumed her position on her back.

"Would you mind taking the watch off for now?" I asked calmly, raising my eyebrows.

She resisted. "I promise, it should be good now. Everyone knows I am in this appointment so they shouldn't bother me."

I began examining her hip, the source of her chronic pain. She winced slightly as I pressed on a tender spot on the side of her hip bone. "It's not just my hip," she admitted, rubbing the back of her neck. "I get these headaches, too. They're almost as bad."

Laying her leg down on the table, I queried, "Did you want to concentrate on the neck or hip today?"

"I don't know. What do you think?" she asked.

"It's really up to you." I paused hoping she would make a decision. But nothing.

"Are the headaches tied to your menstrual cycle?" I was trying to piece together the puzzle.

"Sometimes," she said with a sigh. "But not always. It's like the pain has a mind of its own."

As she spoke, her phone buzzed again from her purse. Her head turned and her eyes darted in the direction of her bag. "Sorry, I don't know who that could be."

Jennifer rolled over and grabbed her phone out of her bag. She glanced at the screen, and while holding her index finger up in the air, she looked back at me sheepishly, replying, "I really need to take this."

The conversation started with, "Hey, I told you I was . . ." and her voice trailed off as she listened intently, eyes darting from left to right continuously.

I watched, feeling a mix of sympathy and irritation as she juggled the call; her stress and now mine was palpable.

She was on the phone for several minutes, her voice a sharp contrast to the soothing environment of the clinic. Our time was slipping away, and I hadn't finished my assessment or started any treatment.

She walked slowly toward my desk, phone to her ear. And then she sat back in the original chair where our conversation started. After a few minutes, I sat behind my desk and as my fingers clicked away on my keyboard as she gave me an apologetic look, mouthing, "I'm sorry," and pointing to her phone.

I glanced at the clock and then back at her, trying to hide my frustration. "We'll need to reschedule," I whispered.

She nodded, her face flushed red as she hurriedly put on her shoes with one hand and straightened her clothes. I opened the door, stepping aside as she walked out.

After she left, I turned to my front office manager. "Next time, she will need to schedule a full evaluation, pay in advance, and promise to turn off her devices," I instructed.

Stephanie, my office manager, nodded.

It was about two weeks later when Stephanie informed me that Jennifer had called back, desperation clear in her voice. The pain she was having was the "worst it has ever been." She scheduled and paid immediately, pledging to disconnect entirely during her visit. As I prepared for her return, I couldn't help but wonder if her alternating hip pain and headaches were merely physical symptoms of the relentless stress she carried; a silent burden that technology and responsibility only seemed to exacerbate.

Cortisol: How Our Stress Hormone Contributes to Pain

Though Jennifer's situation is extreme, it's not that uncommon. The pull of our devices holding a vast reserve of information and responsibilities, literally sitting in front of us or in our pockets or purses all day long, have added to our stress levels.

While there are nearly 8 billion people in the world, at the time of this writing there are 6.5 billion cell phone users. And according to David Greenfield, professor of clinical psychiatry at the University of Connecticut School of Medicine and founder of the Center for Internet and Technology Addiction, "Your cortisol levels are elevated when your phone is in sight and nearby when you hear it or even think you hear it."

With Jennifer, we can see that not only was her phone contributing to her likely elevated cortisol levels, but her current job situation and how she was managing it was undoubtedly causing elevated stress hormones.

Cortisol: The Stress Hormone

You may recall that we briefly discussed cortisol in Chapter 11. It is indeed a hormone, and in our city analogy, cortisol represents our emergency response system. It comes from our adrenal glands that sit on top of each kidney. These adrenal glands have the important job of helping us manage our stress by releasing many different hormones. Cortisol is the one that most people hear about.

Back in the caveman and cavewoman days, when our ancestors were being chased by predators like lions or tigers, we either got eaten, fought, or ran away to survive. Our bodies helped us address these situations by activating our emergency response system and sending signals from the brain to our muscles and organs when we sense danger, which protects us.

As a result of the danger, the adrenals are stimulated and cortisol begins coursing through the body, stimulating muscles to react to either fight or run as fast as possible, potentially up a tree and hopefully out of danger. During this time, the brain switches from trying to understand, i.e., using our executive functioning (planning, organizing, controlling responses) to our reactive brain. The reactive center of our brain, our hindbrain, helps us function quickly without 'thinking.' When a predator is in pursuit, and it is considering you as its next meal; it's not time to contemplate how the tiger got its stripes or whether the lion's name could be Simba. When we are in a dangerous situation, we want our brain and body to take charge and help us get the heck out of Dodge or fight off our attacker.

While this is happening, other organ systems such as the digestive and the reproductive system slow down. Less blood flow is traveling to those organs, while more blood flow travels to the muscles in our extremities. All hands-on deck are necessary to get away from the threat. This also isn't a time to digest our last meal or make babies.

Once this situation escalates, there are only two eventual outcomes. Escape death by killing the predator or getting out of its reach or succumb to the attack and become dinner.

When our ancestors were successful in avoiding their demise, their bodies likely had time to rebalance, whether on the long walk back to the tribe or hanging out up in the tree that saved them. At that time, hormones like cortisol and adrenaline returned to normal, and we went back to the cave or kept on hunting and gathering.

Fast forward to our modern-day world. Hopefully, no tigers are chasing us, but instead, we are dealing with stress in many different ways:

- At work
- In relationships (romantic, family, friends)
- From financial problems
- _____ I am sure you can fill in the blank

Our body doesn't differentiate between the stress we experienced when a tiger was chasing us, when our boss is putting pressure on to hit a deadline, or when our child is in danger. The same response happens to varying degrees.

And these days, it's clear that stress from unrelenting exposure to the constant stimulation of our gadgets, which have become an integral part of our lives, is palpable and creating higher anxiety (aka physiological and emotional stress) levels than we have ever experienced before.

My guess is that you have at least one of these devices within reach right now:

- Smartphones
- Smartwatches
- Other wearable devices that are constantly sending us data and alerts
- The barrage of addicting social media platforms on our phones or laptops

I swore in 2006, when I purchased my first smartphone, that I would not be a slave to its constant demands. Fast forward decades later, and I find myself worrying if I don't know where I put my device. Everything that runs my life lives in the three-by-six-inch little instrument that is typically within arm's reach, or is at least in the same room as I am 24/7.

This microstimulation multiple times a day, in addition to the larger stressful events, can add up and take its toll on our body in many ways.

For example, in their book *The Microstress Effect*, Rob Cross and

Karen Dillon report that microstressors:

1. **Drain personal capacity:** These stressors sap your energy and focus. Examples include unexpected work demands, interruptions, and managing multiple tasks simultaneously.

2. **Deplete emotional reserves:** These stressors affect emotional well-being and can stem from conflicts, misunderstandings, and negative social interactions.

3. **Challenge your identity:** These stressors make you question your values, self-worth, or the meaning of your work. They can arise from situations where your work or actions don't align with your personal values or identity.

In addition to the consequences listed above, these tiny chinks in our stress threshold armor also effect cortisol over time, causing levels to stay elevated. The body's systems were not meant to sustain elevated cortisol for long periods of time. Cortisol is catabolic, meaning it breaks down other molecules. If this action is continuous, it can be detrimental over time. Elevated cortisol levels can lead to persistent fatigue and eventually exhaustion.

Cortisol, Progesterone, and Testosterone

In Chapter 11, we discussed the sex/steroid hormones and how each affects the other in its pathway. When you take another look at those pathways, you see there is a close relationship between cortisol and progesterone in both men and women. Here is the hormone cascade one more time. Note the shaded hormones in this image.

Hormone Pathways

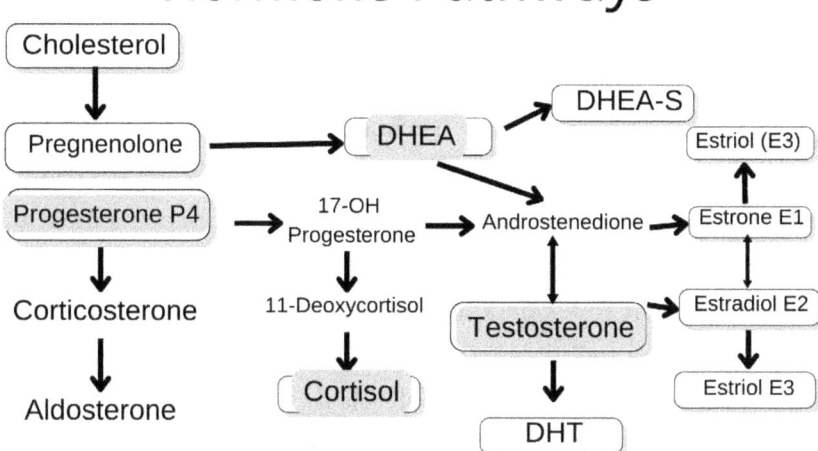

Figure 12.1 Hormone Pathways

The hormone cascade shows a direct relationship between cortisol and progesterone. With continued elevated levels of cortisol, progesterone can be converted to cortisol to make sure we have enough to address that stress. Overtime this can deplete progesterone needed for a woman's menstrual cycle, fertility, or general wellbeing. In men, if elevated cortisol depletes their levels of progesterone, then testosterone levels can fall as well. In both men and women, when cortisol levels remain elevated this typically causes DHEA (considered our anti-aging hormone) to be suppressed over time, contributing to accelerated inflammation. Therefore, the stress response if prolonged can significantly affect our hormones.

Hormone replacement of low progesterone, DHEA or testosterone in situations where someone has been under significant stress and experiencing elevated levels of cortisol and lower levels of DHEA is not addressing the underlying issue. The root cause of the hormone imbalance in these cases is either emotional stress that effects our physiology or physiological stress from what we are putting in or on our body (ultra-processed foods, chemicals, etc).

How Does Cortisol and Subsequently Long-Term Stress Affect the Joints and Muscles?

In a study examining the relationship between cortisol levels and various types of pain—acute, chronic (such as degenerative low back pain), or intermittent (comes and goes, e.g., headaches)—researchers compared the cortisol levels in the blood of participants experiencing muscle and joint pain to those of healthy controls. The cortisol levels were measured at four different times over a twenty-four-hour period. The findings revealed that individuals with intermittent pain exhibited the most significant fluctuations in cortisol levels throughout the day, compared to the other groups and the healthy controls.

In another study looking at women with osteoarthritis in the knee, their pain was related to higher levels of cortisol when observed by taking cortisol samples four times per day. The cortisol levels increased when pain levels were higher.

Therefore, when our stress levels are high, our pain and potentially inflammation can be exacerbated. Or our pain contributes to our stress. It can be a vicious cycle.

I Carry My Stress Here

It's relatively common to hear people say, "I carry my stress here," as they are grabbing and massaging their upper trapezius muscles that sit on their shoulders. Why do those muscles become painful?

In Chapter 11, I also discussed how the thyroid gland can be an issue when you have aching muscles, but cortisol can affect the muscles, as well. Remember, cortisol is the fight, flight, or freeze hormone. So, when cortisol is elevated, more blood is going to the muscles. But in modern times when we don't have the opportunity to fight or flee. Therefore, these muscles can remain constantly stimulated by cortisol and remain upregulated or on guard, eventually leading to decreased blood flow to the area. This results in increased tension or that hard feeling you get when you feel your muscle and it feels really tight. Massage, acupuncture, electrical stimulation, and other modalities such as SoftWave can help relax these muscles by bringing blood flow to the area immediately. Exercise is also beneficial, as the pumping mechanism of the muscle causes it to contract and relax, helping to release tension and pump new blood into the area. But if stress is not addressed, the relief from exercise and modalities is typically short-lived, thus leading to feeling as if we hold our stress in various muscles in the body.

Pain at Night

Both low and high cortisol can contribute to muscle and joint pain. As we discussed, high cortisol can be associated with increased pain.

But it doesn't only cause problems if it's too high. In addition to being one of the hormones in our emergency response system, when cortisol is balanced it also keeps the immune system from becoming overaggressive. In our city (the body), while cortisol is often seen rushing to crises (stressful events), it also has a critical role in keeping the city's maintenance workers (immune system) in check, preventing them from causing unnecessary damage (inflammation) when making repairs. The cortisol we make in our body, when called upon under normal circumstances, helps assist in repair of the body. It has a potent, natural anti-inflammatory effect.

> You may have heard of someone taking cortisone or drugs called corticosteroids like prednisone. They are derivatives of cortisol and can have a potent systemic anti-inflammatory effect by shutting down the inflammation process. These levels are consistently much higher than the levels our body would naturally make.

Long-term use of these medications can cause a myriad of health issues like osteoporosis, osteonecrosis (death of bones), muscle wasting, diabetes, infections, and more, so they should be monitored appropriately, and you should have the goal of taking the least amount possible to minimize risk.

Due to this anti-inflammatory effect, our body's natural production of cortisol helps to keep pain from conditions such as arthritis at bay.

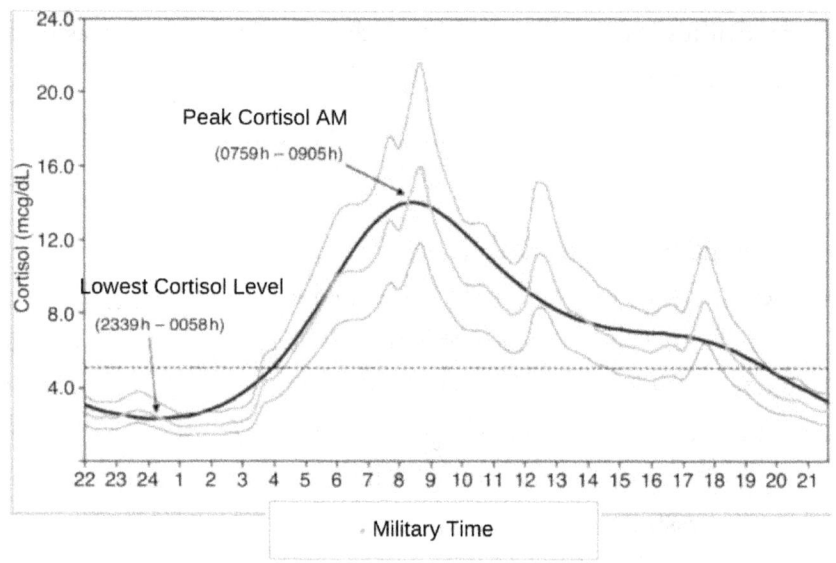

Figure 12.2 Diurnal cortisol pattern; cortisol is highest in the morning, then decreases before bed to allow sleep.

But cortisol doesn't just stay at one level throughout the day. It fluctuates and exhibits what is referred to as a diurnal pattern. See Figure 12.2. Cortisol should be higher in the morning hours to help us wake up and have enough energy during the day. When cortisol is too low or too high at night or even during the day, this can cause the joints to ache. One reason why cortisol lowers naturally at night is so that its stimulus doesn't keep us awake or doesn't wake us up during the night.

Serotonin: How a Mood Regulator Can Impact Joint and Muscle Pain

It's not uncommon today to struggle with mental health issues. A 2023 Gallup poll out of Washington, D.C., showed that "the percentage of US adults who report having been diagnosed with depression at some point in their lifetime has reached 29 percent, nearly 10 percentage points higher than in 2015."

Many have heard or read about the neurotransmitter serotonin being associated with depression and the target of many antidepressants classified as selective serotonin reuptake inhibitors (SSRIs). But how could our body's naturally occurring serotonin be associated with joint or muscle pain?

Let's define what a neurotransmitter such as serotonin is, what it does, and how it travels. We've built quite an analogy with the body and its systems functioning as a city and its inhabitants.

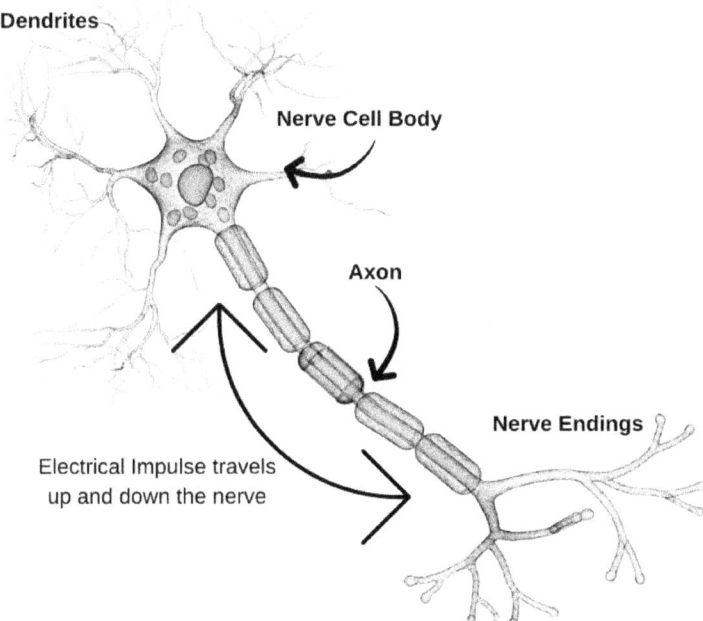

Figure 12.3: This image depicts a neuron/nerve, highlighting its key components: the nerve cell body, dendrites, axon, and nerve endings. The diagram shows the pathway of electrical impulses traveling from the dendrites through the axon to the nerve endings.

Neurons or nerve cells travel throughout our body carrying signals by an innate electrical system. See Figure 12.3.

According to *Scientific American*, in the brain alone there are 86 billion neurons. The digestive system, including the gut, has 100 million neurons as well, all connecting pathways back to the brain and spinal cord. This essentially is what landline telephone cables used to do from house to house. These landlines were once essential for communication, carrying signals and connecting various parts of the city. In our body think of those various parts as the brain, gut, and the rest of the organs and tissues in the body.

Neurotransmitters, such as serotonin, are akin to the signals exchanged at the telephone poles. Once the exchange takes place at the telephone pole, the signal continues along the wire to the next pole and continues to its destination. In the body, between nerves there are spaces called synapses. Think of these synapses as a space at the telephone poll where one signal jumps to the next cable. In our neurological system, neurotransmitters are the chemicals released into these synapses to continue, stop, speed up, or potentially slow down the signal from the brain and spinal cord to its final destination. In other words, at the junction of the cable and the telephone poles (the synapse), the signals create a reaction (neurotransmitters) that facilitates the transmission of signals between landlines (neurons).

In the brain, serotonin helps regulate mood, anxiety, and happiness. But its influence extends far beyond just how we feel emotionally. Serotonin is also found in the gut. As a matter of fact, 95 percent of the body's production of serotonin occurs in the gut, not the brain. Another reason to optimize gut health when it comes to pain, as you will see.

Serotonin Can Increase or Decrease Pain

Pain is a complex experience that involves sensory, emotional, and cognitive components. Serotonin contributes to pain modulation by influencing the pain pathways in the central nervous system (the brain and spinal cord) and gut. It can both inhibit and facilitate pain, depending on the receptors it activates and the areas of the brain, spinal cord, and gut it affects.

1. **Inhibitory Role:** Serotonin can activate certain receptors that inhibit the transmission of pain signals, effectively reducing pain perception. This is why some medications that increase serotonin levels are used to treat chronic pain conditions.

2. **Facilitatory Role:** Conversely, serotonin can also enhance pain perception under certain circumstances. This dual role is due to the presence of different types of serotonin receptors throughout the body, each with distinct functions. That is why these same medications can contribute to muscle and joint pain in some people.

It is clear in the research that prolonged stress is associated with low serotonin levels. If these neurotransmitter levels are low due to significant emotional and/or physiological stressors, increased pain can ensue.

In some cases, managing moods by manipulating serotonin with selective serotonin reuptake inhibitors (SSRI's) can also contribute to muscle and joint pain. Though these medications can be lifesaving at times, it is important to consider them as a source of muscle or joint pain.

> Suzie came to see me in the clinic for upper back pain. She was nineteen and had struggled emotionally in her first year of college, so her doctor put her on a popular SSRI. Suzie and her mother came to me to discuss her upper back pain. They had tried everything: physical therapy, other exercise, acupuncture, and chiropractic care, but nothing seemed to work. Her doctor had mentioned that they could try Botox injections, but she did not want to pursue that option.
>
> Whenever I see patients, I always review their supplements and medications. I asked Suzie when her pain had started, and she said it had been approximately six months prior. When I asked her when she started the SSRI, she said it was

seven months before. As Suzie answered that question, she and her mom both looked at each other and then back at me. "Do you think the medication could be causing the pain?" they asked.

I replied by saying muscle and joint pain was a potential side effect of that medication.

"Should I come off of it?" Suzie asked, after first glancing back at her mom.

"That is something you and your provider should discuss. You never want to stop these medications without weaning off of them, so if you do decide to stop or change medications, please consult with your provider before doing so. You may also want to consider seeing a therapist for cognitive behavior therapy," I suggested, "to help you through the difficult transition to college. In addition, there may be other medications that you could try with the guidance of your provider."

Next, I explained what would happen in our treatments and we talked about SoftWave as a potential modality. Suzie and her mom decided to hold off on pursuing the treatment at our clinic and instead wanted to consult her physician about the medication. When my office manager called Suzie four weeks later to see how she was doing, she let us know she no longer had the upper back pain after weaning off of the medication with the guidance of her physician, and she was seeing her therapist again.

More Neurotransmitters and Hormones Impact Pain

Chronic pain conditions, such as fibromyalgia, a condition where several trigger points of pain are found in many muscles around the body, are often associated with central sensitization, where the central nervous system (brain and spinal cord) becomes hypersensitive to pain stimuli. It is thought that low serotonin levels can contribute to this heightened sensitivity, making individuals more prone to experiencing pain from stimuli that would not normally be painful. For example, it has been reported that patients with fibromyalgia often have lower levels of serotonin, which is thought to contribute to their widespread pain and increased pain sensitivity.

Interestingly enough, estrogen impacts the making of serotonin by influencing the production of another neurotransmitter called tryptophan. Tryptophan converts into serotonin. And when estrogen is present, tryptophan can increase, and so does the amount of serotonin present. Studies dating back to 1993 showed this correlation. So, one can surmise that as estrogen levels decrease in menopause, potentially serotonin decreases as well.

In addition, studies have also shown that cortisol, both elevated and low, can lower tryptophan production, thus affecting the amount of serotonin available and could be another reason why stress, causing low serotonin, contributes to increased pain.

As I have mentioned, serotonin is also crucial for mood regulation. Depression and anxiety, which are linked to low serotonin levels, are related to exacerbating the perception of pain. This connection creates a cycle where pain worsens mood, and poor mood increases pain perception. For example, individuals with chronic depression often report higher levels of muscle and joint pain. It's a vicious cycle.

There is a delicate dance that hormones and neurotransmitters are engaged in. Suffice it to say, the balance is complex and intricate, and stress impacts this balance, which in turn can impact pain.

Melatonin and Serotonin Relationship: Another Link to Pain

Most people are likely aware that not getting enough sleep can impact their energy levels and behaviors. The body needs its time to rest and recuperate.

One of the hormones helping to regulate sleep is melatonin. As darkness falls and less light hits the retina of our eyes, the pineal gland in the brain secretes melatonin to begin our natural progression towards sleep.

Melatonin can then be considered the night watchman of our city. In historical and modern contexts, night watchmen patrol premises, buildings, or areas to ensure that everything is secure, checking for any signs of trouble, and responding to emergencies. They play a crucial role in safeguarding property and people during the hours when most are asleep, ensuring that any disturbances or issues are addressed promptly to maintain safety and peace. Getting enough sleep will help melatonin assist the body, just like the night watchman helps the city stay peaceful.

- **Signaling the Transition to Night**: Just as a night watchman begins their shift when the day ends, melatonin levels rise as daylight fades, signaling to the body that it's time to prepare for sleep.
- **Inducing Sleepiness**: The night watchman ensures that everyone in the city (the body) knows it's time to rest. Melatonin promotes feelings of sleepiness and helps the body transition into sleep mode.
- **Maintaining a Regular Schedule**: The night watchman helps the city keep to regular nighttime routine. The same is true for melatonin as it helps to ensure that the body's internal clock stays on track, which is essential for maintaining a consistent sleep-wake cycle.
- **Ensuring Quality Rest**: By keeping the city calm and quiet, the night watchman (melatonin) ensures that the city's residents (the body's systems) get the rest they need to function optimally the next day.

When you don't get enough sleep, this effects important hormones in your body that usually help reduce pain, one of them being melatonin. This hormone has been proven to be a natural analgesic or pain reducer. On the flip side, lack of sleep makes other systems more active, like those that cause inflammation and an increase in pain signals.

Some people report pain keeps them up or disturbs their sleep. In addition, lack of sleep itself can make pain worse, whether it's acute pain or long-term pain.

And here's another interesting tidbit: guess what neurotransmitter makes melatonin? There's that serotonin again! The relationship is also complex. While melatonin rises to put you to sleep and falls as we get closer to waking; serotonin rises along with cortisol as we begin coming out of our slumber. I always remember this relationship with this phrase: Mel puts you to bed, and Sera wakes you up in the morning.

Knowing that fact, you can probably surmise that if the body is low in serotonin, then you may not have the melatonin you need to get a good night's sleep to help your body and mind address pain.

Jennifer, the healthcare CEO we met earlier who was chained to her devices, was released from her position when the hospital was bought out by a larger system. She was lucky enough to receive a severance package, so she did not have to start work right away. When she returned to the clinic after six months in her forced retirement, she was a different person. The first thing I noticed was the absence of her Apple Watch. In its place was a simple wristband that only tracked her heart rate, body temperature, and sleep patterns. She smiled as she explained that after leaving her job, the constant tension in her neck and the relentless headaches had finally subsided. While she wasn't yet getting a full eight hours of sleep each night, she proudly told me she was consistently managing seven hours—and her phone now lived on the kitchen counter, far from her bed.

We focused on her hip pain during her sessions, and after just three treatments of SoftWave therapy, combined with manual therapy, exercise, and a few adjustments to her shoe orthotics, Jennifer was pain-free. She was even excited to share that she had tried paddleboarding for the first time, something she never had time to do before.

Jennifer's experience highlights the profound impact that stress has on our bodies. While you may not be able to put a hold on your career or job to address your stress, managing stress is crucial to optimizing hormone levels, gut health, and ultimately reducing inflammation, which is a significant contributor to chronic pain.

How Do You Manage Stress?

I think we all know what we are supposed to do to address stress.

Meditation, yoga, physical exercise, mindfulness, and even breathing exercises have hundreds, if not thousands of research studies now to support their beneficial effects on our hormones, our gut health, and our stress levels. All of these are helpful to address pain, as well.

But what I will challenge you to do is to not beat yourself up for what you aren't doing—but instead to examine what you *are* doing and see if it is helping or hurting you.

What are your current stress-management strategies? You may tell me that you don't have one or any, but my guess is you do have one, if not several ways that you are managing your stress, but they may not be the most effective or helpful for your system.

Here are the most common stress-management strategies that I see my patients participating in that are likely contributing to inflammation and pain.

- Alcohol consumption
- Overeating
- Eating foods that taste good, but you know aren't great for you
- Scrolling on your phone first thing in the morning, last thing before going to bed at night, at stop lights, in traffic, and whenever there is downtime
- Watching hours of television

- Overexercising (pushing yourself to exercise even though you are exhausted, and it hurts)
- Avoiding all exercise due to anticipating pain, or you don't have time
- Less common these days is smoking cigarettes (thank goodness)

I am not saying these are all bad and you should never partake in any of them (except smoking, that's a hard no). Believe me, I binge watch a good show with the best of them. But if you can check off two, three, or more of the stress management techniques on this list, then you are likely contributing to less-than-optimal gut health and hormone levels while ramping up inflammation that could be contributing to your pain.

And here's the best part. You can do something about it.

How?

Well, ... one step at a time.

Take one of the inflammation-contributing strategies from the list, or any other one that you know you are currently taking part in, and switch it out for one of the following.

Eating Plan

Research the Mediterranean diet and change one or two meals a week to eating this way, and then increase the frequency of healthy foods over time.

- Decrease sugar and allow yourself a "treat" once or twice a week.
- Stick to the foods you know you don't react to or do the ALCAT test to find what your body is reacting to and what it isn't.
- Pick one day a week to do food prep.
- Find a nonalcoholic healthy beverage to drink besides water (Beware: zero sugar usually means artificial sweeteners, which you typically want to avoid).

Exercise

- If you are exhausted most of the time, choose restorative exercises like yoga and get your hormones checked.
- Find a pool near you and walk, swim, or join a class.
- Do your exercises within non-painful range, even if it's just for five mins a day and very small movements. You have to start somewhere. Or find a personal trainer or physical therapist to help guide you.
- Practice mindfulness by taking a walk if you can without listening to anything, and just enjoying the outdoors.
- Find yoga poses that contribute to relief and help you relax.
- Discover your healthy heart zones to exercise within (at our clinic we measure patients resting and active metabolic rates to determine these) and commit to working up to thirty minutes or more each time you exercise.

Socializing

- Find a nonalcoholic, healthy beverage that you can enjoy out with friends (Beware: zero sugar usually means artificial sweeteners which you typically want to avoid).
- Watch an uplifting movie or comedienne with friends.
- Take a walk with people you enjoy being with.
- Give a friend who tends to brighten your mood a call.

Managing Media

- Put your phone in the other room to charge overnight if possible.
- Keep your phone in your purse, pocket, or bag while you are in the car.
- Listen to your favorite songs or inspirational fun podcasts while driving.
- Read or listen to a book that will help you move closer to a goal in your life.

Mind Body/Brain Body Time

- Meditation
- Visualization
- Prayer
- Mindfulness activities

This list is definitely not complete, but start switching out one or two things a week to do consistently or rotate some of the above, whatever works for you.

There are many other healthy stress-management techniques you can partake in. Try some out from our list and create your own. The trick is to believe you are important enough to make these changes and implement them.

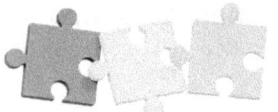

Key Pieces

Stress and Pain Connection: Chronic stress can significantly contribute to physical pain. In addition, pain exacerbates chronic stress.

Cortisol's Role: Elevated or low cortisol levels, triggered by ongoing stress, can increase pain and inflammation in the body and can affect other hormones such as progesterone, testosterone, and DHEA. Over time, this can lead to fatigue and exacerbate pain.

Neurotransmitters and Hormones: Stress impacts serotonin, a neurotransmitter that regulates mood and pain. It can both inhibit and facilitate pain depending on its levels and the receptors it activates. Low serotonin, often linked to stress and poor mental health, can contribute to increased pain sensitivity and chronic pain conditions. In addition, low serotonin may contribute to low melatonin levels, negatively impacting sleep and potentially intensifying pain. Keep in mind that a lack of sleep can exacerbate pain.

Healthy Stress Management: Developing effective stress-management strategies is essential in optimizing cortisol, serotonin, and melatonin levels to alleviate pain. Avoiding harmful stress management techniques like overconsumption of alcohol, smoking, or unhealthy foods is crucial.

CHAPTER 13

The Brain and Your Pain

"Pain is clearly in your body, but 100 percent of the time without exception it's produced by your brain."

–Author Lorimer Moseley

Don arrived early for his appointment, stepping into the clinic with an air of casual confidence. He wore a light blue golfer's polo top and blue jeans, complemented by pristine white tennis shoes that gleamed without a scuff. As he settled into the chair opposite me, he smiled warmly, but the slight tension in his eyes hinted at the discomfort he was experiencing.

"Good morning, Don," I greeted him. "How are you today?"

"I'm doing well, thank you," Don replied. "But obviously I could be better."

I glanced at his questionnaire on my laptop. "Yes, it says here you are having problems with your back and occasionally your legs," I confirmed.

"That's right," he said. He reached around his left side. "It is really starting to affect my golf game."

"Do you have pain while playing golf?" I asked.

"Sometimes," he responded. "Sometimes, I will get a sharp pain when I move a certain way." Don rotated his torso in his seat, his face wincing slightly. "But most of the time it is sore a couple hours after I play golf and sometimes tight and uncomfortable before I start."

"Does anything reduce the pain?" I asked.

Donald went on, "When I hit some balls to warm up, it helps, but I feel like my motion is limited when I try to swing, even when I am not experiencing pain."

He described his condition, mentioning that the pain would "come and go," occasionally "shooting down" one of his legs. "I work in finance, and normally I sit a lot," he explained. "As I'm nearing retirement though, I've been playing more golf, which I love. But this back pain is really getting in the way."

I nodded and found myself adjusting my posture. "Tell me more about your other activities," I encouraged.

"Well, aside from golf, I've started cycling alongside my son while he is running," Don said, as a smile spread across his face. "He's training for a marathon, and I'm hoping to run alongside him while he trains to encourage him." His eyes lit up. "I used to be an avid runner when I was younger. And being active with him makes me realize how much I miss it."

As Don spoke, he sat up in his chair and scooted toward my desk, gently tapping his fist while describing how proud he was of his son and how participating in his training helped him feel as though they were growing closer. "And besides spending time with him, it's motivating me to get this back taken care of so I can stay active when I retire in twelve months. I have had this on and off now for probably two years. It was better and now it's getting worse again."

"I understand how frustrating this must be for you," I said. "What did you do before to address the pain?"

"Have you heard of Dr. John Sarno?" he asked, with a slightly strained look on his face.

I smiled and responded, "Yes, he wrote the book *Healing Your Back*."

Donald's shoulders began to relax, and the tension left his face. "His information helped me a lot. It was the first time that I heard about how to address pain that did not go away. Dr. Sarno's approach really changed the way I thought about the pain I had." He continued, "Most of my providers either haven't heard of him or don't believe his system works. But it worked for me." He paused. "But now I feel like I need a bit more help."

It was wonderful to hear that a patient was talking about an approach that was very different (yet effective) from the way chronic pain is normally treated in the conventional medical system.

As we continued our conversation and discussed treatment options, the room filled with a sense of optimism and determination. I knew that, like many of my patients, he was motivated to address his pain, but the fact that he was familiar with different concepts of what causes and contributes to chronic pain made me even more optimistic. I had a feeling he would understand the concept of intangible triggers that are addressed in this book. Current research about pain science and chronic pain often discuss intangible triggers that can't easily be seen or measured.

As I do with all my patients, I asked Don what else in the past or present he had done to help with his pain. He recited a long list: physical therapy, massage, chiropractic treatments, but he said the thing that helped him most was addressing his belief about his pain. During our time together, Don shared his story.

When MRI Findings Don't Tell the Whole Story

Don took me back to his experience with his first orthopedic physicians. He had been grappling with pain for more than a few months before he sought help; a period long enough for his condition to be classified as chronic pain. Two MRIs—one ordered by his orthopedic surgeon and another he sought independently—revealed disc bulges. However, the findings weren't significant enough to warrant surgery. His physician explained that many people Don's age have similar changes in their spines without experiencing any pain, suggesting that fixing these areas surgically often doesn't lead to improvement.

In fact, as early as 1994, a study published in *The New England Journal of Medicine* highlighted that many individuals who had no pain at all showed disc bulges or disc protrusions on MRI. The researchers concluded, "Given the high prevalence of these findings and of back pain, the discovery by MRI of bulges or protrusions in people with low back pain may frequently be coincidental."

This indicates that MRI findings may not always correlate with the source of the pain.

Since he wasn't convinced the MRI findings were relevant, Don's surgeon referred Don to physical therapy, which provided some relief. However, upon further discussion, it became clear that Don's therapy sessions were largely exercise-based, with zero hands-on treatment. The busy clinic environment meant his therapist was often juggling multiple patients at once, leaving Don feeling that he could just as easily do the exercises at home.

A Note on Physical Therapy

If you find that your physical therapy sessions consist solely of exercises without any hands-on treatment, consider finding another clinic. Due to decreased reimbursement from insurance companies, many large practices are forced to pack in patients, turning physical therapists into solely exercise instructors rather than allowing them to work to the full extent of their license. Effective patient care should include one-on-one time, movement and biomechanics assessment, appropriate manual therapy, and ideally, advanced treatments like SoftWave therapy.

Exploring Beyond the MRI

Don's understanding of the MRI findings and the limited success of physical therapy led him to investigate other potential causes for his persistent pain. He recalled a minor injury from twisting the wrong way years ago, but he felt that should have resolved by now. He also considered his history of running in his teens and twenties but noted that many of his friends continued to run into their forties and fifties without experiencing back pain.

Determined to find answers, Don explored the possibility that factors beyond physical abnormalities were contributing to his chronic pain. What he discovered was life-changing.

Diving deep into Doctor Google territory, Don scrolled upon the work of Dr. John Sarno, a pioneering orthopedic surgeon, physician, and professor of rehabilitation medicine who developed a novel approach to understanding and treating chronic back pain. After years of doing surgery on thousands of patients with back pain, Dr. Sarno grew increasingly frustrated that after 'fixing' anatomically what he found was wrong on MRIs and during surgery patient's symptoms were the same or worse after their surgeries. So Sarno began to explore what else could be causing the ongoing, often severe, pain. Surprisingly, he stumbled on the connection between emotions and physical pain. Dr. Sarno wrote about this connection and how it completely changed the way he treated his patients in his book *Healing Back Pain*. Don devoured the book and began to understand the principles behind the doctor's success with patients.

Here is a summary of Dr. Sarno's concepts related to what he coined, the Mindbody Syndrome:

Mindbody Syndrome (TMS)

- **Theory**: Dr. Sarno proposed that many cases of chronic back pain are caused by tension myositis syndrome (TMS), which he later referred to as 'mindbody syndrome.' He believed that the pain is not due to structural abnormalities, but rather emotional and psychological factors.
- **Emotional Causes**: According to Sarno, repressed emotions such as anger, anxiety, and stress lead to physical symptoms. The brain, in an effort to protect the individual from facing these uncomfortable emotions, diverts attention by creating pain in the body.
- **Psychosomatic Response**: Sarno argued that the subconscious mind induces muscle tension and reduced blood flow to certain areas, resulting in pain and other symptoms. This is Sarno's argument, but it hasn't been substantiated in research. Pain hypersensitivity, discussed later, has been substantiated through research. This doesn't lessen Sarno's argument, as his would be an example of an intangible trigger, since the subconscious mind can't be measured. However, the changes in the brain due to neuroplasticity can be measured, albeit not easily.

Diagnosis and Treatment

- **Diagnosis**: Sarno's diagnosis of TMS involved ruling out serious medical conditions through physical examinations and imaging studies. He focused on identifying emotional and psychological stressors in the patient's life.
- **Education**: A crucial part of Sarno's treatment was educating patients about the potential psychological origins of their pain.

He emphasized that understanding and acknowledging the emotional causes of pain could significantly alleviate symptoms.

- **Psychotherapy:** Sarno recommended psychotherapy or counseling for patients to explore and address repressed emotions. Techniques such as journaling and mindfulness were also suggested to help patients process their feelings. He reported case study after case study that showed as patients allowed themselves to feel the repressed emotions of anger, rage, fear or guilt, the patients initially noted increased pain during the treatment, but gradually, as they let those emotions go by working through the root cause, the physical pain either significantly reduced or was eliminated.

- **Outcome:** Thousands of Dr. Sarno's patients reported significant improvements or complete resolution of their pain by following his approach, often after years of suffering and failed traditional treatments.

After reading through the work of Dr. Sarno, Don was convinced that his issues were related to significant stress from work and problems he was having with his relationship. He started to note that any time he felt under pressure and became angry or frustrated about work or his relationship, the pain would increase. In addition, his baseline was constant low-grade pain.

His method to reduce pain was keeping in mind that the problem was not in his back. His back pain was a harbinger that reminded him he wasn't letting go of the built-up emotions connected to his job and his personal life. Instead of taking multiple medications to suppress or cover up the pain, Don realized the pain was his body talking to him, and when it would flare up or he would notice it, he had developed his own routine regarding how to get rid of it.

- First, he would acknowledge that he was aware of the pain and go

to a place where he had little distraction. He might find himself going to his car, a spare room, or even the bathroom.
- Next, he would remind himself that the pain was not physical pain, but instead a result of his current or past emotional state.
- And finally, he would practice diaphragmatic breathing to slow down his body's stress response, continue repeating to himself that his pain was not in his back, but instead in his brain, and low and behold, his pain would slowly go away.

Don admitted, "The first time I went through these steps, I felt really uncomfortable. My conscious mind seemed to be fighting me at the beginning, telling me, 'This is ridiculous. This is stupid. Your pain is in your back. It's from the discs, etc, etc.' But a funny thing happened when I said those things to myself: I noticed the pain actually increased. This told me it did have to do with my brain more than my body, because I wasn't doing anything at the time except for running these comments through my head, so it couldn't have been caused by anything physical in that moment."

Was Don just convincing himself that this was working? Was this simply a placebo effect where he thought it was going to help, and so it did?

The Research About Chronic Pain and the Brain

It is imperative that society and clinicians stop thinking about chronic pain as merely a prolonged version of acute pain. Why? Because research shows that there are many potential causes. It is time for patients and professionals alike to understand that the experience of chronic pain in the body can result in significant alterations in the brain's structure and function. Yes, that is correct: changes in the brain and its interpretation of pain can happen when you suffer with chronic pain. This doesn't mean you are making up your pain, but it does mean that some or all of your pain may be coming from the changes in your brain versus the tissues of an original injury or just from wear and tear.

This research has been gaining ground for decades but is rarely, if ever, applied in the clinical setting. Healthcare practitioners a) don't believe it, or b) have experienced their patient's negative responses when you tell them that the pain is 'in their head.' This stems from years of the medical profession telling patients who continued to experience pain despite surgery or other treatments that their pain was essentially made up. They were and still are told there is nothing physically wrong with them, *or* they are told that there are structural issues as seen on diagnostic tests, but the only answers are medications that, by the way, can make the pain worse in the long run.

In the past, these medical professionals were correct, but not in the way they intended. Research shows that, indeed, pain is in the patient's head. That is, the pain is in the brain.

The City's Districts

Let's go back to our city analogy. This time let's refer to the brain as its own large metropolitan hub. Think of the largest cities in the world sitting inside your head. Relevant brain structures can be seen in Figure 13.1.

- **The Prefrontal Cortex** is the city government headquarters. It's where critical decisions are made, policies are created, and emotional regulations are enforced.
- **The Amygdala** is the city's emergency response center, processing and reacting to emotional alarms and stress signals.
- **The Hippocampus** serves as the city's library and archives, storing memories and helping the citizens recall past events.

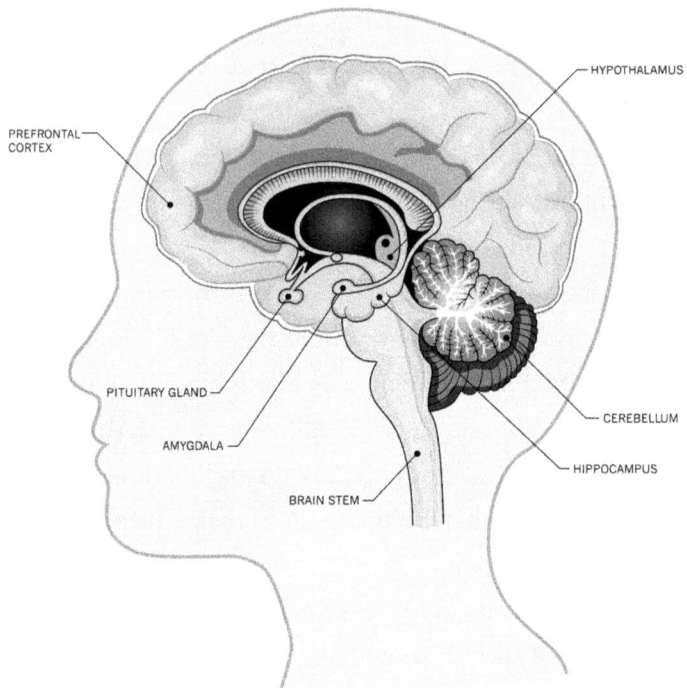

Figure 13.1 Brain Structures

Chronic Pain: The Ongoing Construction

When chronic pain invades the city, it's like an unplanned and prolonged construction project in areas that are vital to everyday activities, including the city center/government buildings (prefrontal cortex).

Chronic pain disrupts the normal flow and function in those areas. The budget keeps getting renewed for this never-ending construction project (chronic pain). It seems like the workers are repeating the same work day in and day out (repetitive thoughts, feelings, and beliefs about pain). Therefore, the neurons related to pain in the brain continue to fire together and wire together, reinforcing their construction project, i.e. pain.

Ultimately the construction (pain) is trying to help or even protect the city, but its constant presence is very irritating. It reduces the efficiency of the traffic around the area it impacts most (the prefrontal cortex), making traffic (decision-making) and communication (hormone balance related to emotional regulation) more challenging.

The cycle continues.

This continued construction:

- Overworks the emergency response center (the amygdala: responsible for emotional processing and reactions), leading to heightened and prolonged emotional stress (cortisol) responses. Traffic jams, accidents, road rage, and the mess of continued construction take their toll. In the body, this results in pain signals continually being generated and heightened, also affecting our emotional responses.
- The dust and mess clutters the library and archives (the hippocampus), making it harder to store and retrieve memories efficiently. Physically, it becomes harder and harder to remember what life was like without the pain.

Pain Hypersensitivity: Your Brain and Body's Version of Road Rage

Pain hypersensitivity, or hyperalgesia, is a common feature of chronic pain. This occurs when individuals experience heightened pain responses to stimuli that would not ordinarily be painful or not as painful as what they would typically experience.

Imagine this:

You believe you tend to be a normal, calm, and rational person. You pride yourself in keeping your emotions in check. But this constant construction on your way to work is raking on your last nerve and the last nerve of other less-centered individuals traveling around you. You have been sitting in this crazy construction zone day after day, month after month, and sometimes year after year. You sometimes feel that at any moment in the middle of this mess you are going to lose it, and indeed some people do. Have you ever flipped someone off or swore (or really *really* wanted to) at other drivers or at whoever is responsible for the ridiculousness of this constant construction? Enter road rage. For those who experience it, road rage hits when there is a heightened sense of stress, and the aggravation of the same stress-filled situation happens time and time again.

This action of a heightened state of stress and irritation describes pain hypersensitivity.

Signals coming from your brain, spinal cord, and periphery (the rest of your body) repeating for months or even years results in the pain being reinforced, and literally, as discussed, it changes your brain. Pain hypersensitivity is common with chronic pain and is often linked to a concept called central sensitization, a process where the central nervous system becomes more sensitive to stimuli due to repeated or prolonged pain signals. As discussed in Chapter 1, NSAIDs and pain medications such as opioids, when taken long-term, can result in this pain hypersensitivity and central sensitization, as well.

Central sensitization involves changes in the spinal cord and brain that amplify pain signals, making the nervous system more responsive to both painful and non-painful stimuli. This can even lead to neuropathy, where even light touch or mild pressure can cause pain.

The Power of Neuroplasticity and Decreasing Pain Hypersensitivity

Neuroplasticity is the brain's remarkable ability to adapt. Yes, even *your* brain can adapt at your age. In other words, the brain, through neuroplasticity, can reorganize itself by forming new neural connections throughout life. This adaptability allows the brain to compensate for injury, adjust to new experiences, and respond to changes in the environment. However, in the context of chronic pain, neuroplasticity can also lead to maladaptive changes that perpetuate pain and exacerbate symptoms . . . and it can be your ticket to pain relief.

Keeping with our analogy, neuroplasticity is the city's (brain's) infrastructure planning department. In the brain, neuroplasticity is the ability of the brain to adapt and rewire itself in response to these disruptions.

Clearly, the old construction project that never seems to end isn't working (you still have pain). So, it is time to overhaul the department. Gradually let go of the workers (thoughts, beliefs, feelings) who were reinforcing the old construction that was not getting you to where you wanted to go, and hire brand-new, experienced supervisors and workers to clean up the mess and create new routes (neural pathways).

Neuroplasticity creates the new department. It allows the brain to form new neural connections and pathways to detour around old areas that reinforce pain and eventually create new construction that moves away from the pain. It just needs direction and reinforcement, and according to research, it needs to get that direction from you.

How Does Neuroplasticity Work?

- **Building New Roads**: After realizing that the construction zones (chronic pain) were necessary at one point to protect the city (brain) from conditions getting worse, the city (brain) constructs new roads (neural pathways) to reroute traffic and improve connectivity and communication between different districts (brain and body). These messages are simply protective, nudging us to shift our beliefs away from feeling controlled by the pain.

- Understanding these processes helps you understand that you do have influence over the pain's existence and intensity. You don't have to solely rely on something outside of you to get rid of your pain. The result: you can lessen the pain or eliminate it.

- **Renovating Structures**: Even if some buildings (brain regions) are outdated and in need of repair, the city can renovate and repurpose them, enhancing their functionality. Research shows that this happens in the brain. When an area is not functioning as well as it should, another area can, in many cases, take over its function. New area, new thoughts, new beliefs, improved hormone production, and an uptick in the natural pain-relieving substances in our body, such as endorphins, can be released to help address the pain.

- **Improving Communication**: The altered connectivity in the brain's pain processing pathways is like installing new communication networks, putting up new signs for detours, and ensuring that despite the disruptions, the city can still function and process information effectively. Therefore, there is no need for the road rage (pain hypersensitivity) anymore. New roads or neural networks are created. New beliefs about the pain are reinforced and the new neural networks fire together and wire together.

The new project gets underway, and with reinforcement and time, the changes become more permanent.

Hopefully you recognize by now that when you feel the pain in your body somewhere, your perception of that pain is always being created in the brain.

But is this all really true? Is there any proof?

Phantom Limb Pain: Proof that Pain Is Produced in Your Brain

Scientists and clinicians began to realize that pain doesn't always come from the area that hurts when dealing with the phenomenon of phantom pain. This occurs when a person has their limb amputated, but they still feel pain where their limb used to be.

Since their body part is no longer there, how could a person feel pain and perceive that pain to be in the limb that is no longer present? Let's say a person is forty-five when they have their lower leg amputated. For forty-five years, they believed they had a leg there. For forty-five years walking on that leg, kicking a ball with that foot, putting on socks and shoes reinforced the neural pathways in the brain supporting the fact that a leg (and foot) existed. Now, after amputation, suddenly and traumatically, the leg and foot are gone. But the neural networks in the brain created to reinforce the existence of the leg remain.

Cognitive behavioral therapy, a technique called the mirroring exercise, virtual apps, and other exercises have helped those with phantom limb pain reduce or eliminate it. All of these techniques are creating new neural networks in the brain by addressing the thoughts, beliefs, and even the emotions associated with phantom limb pain. Since the patient, in most cases, can look down and see that there is no limb there, these therapies and tools help rewire the unconscious beliefs that a leg and foot still exists as well as address the emotional turmoil that would accompany such a devastating situation.

That is good news!

Since the pain you experience comes from the brain, due to neuroplasticity, it's a fact that the brain can change and so can your pain. It can lessen or even go away.

The brain is not static. It is a dynamic and resilient city, always capable of adapting and reorganizing to maintain its vital functions. This means you can get control over your pain instead of the pain having control over you.

How To Tap Into Neuroplasticity: Steps to Rewire Your Brain's Pain Response

Lorimer Moseley, a prominent pain researcher, has emphasized the importance of pain education in changing patients' beliefs and attitudes about pain. Moseley's research has shown that when his "Explain Pain" approach involves educating patients about the neuroscience of pain, and this education is coupled with physical therapy, exercise or treatment modalities, they achieve better outcomes. Coupling these concepts together is called cognitive functional therapy (CFT). And research is showing that this combination can be very successful.

A study published in the medical journal *The Lancet* reported that "CFT can produce large and sustained improvements for people with chronic disabling low back pain."

In other words, helping patients understand that pain does not always correlate with tissue damage or what is seen on tests such as an MRI, along with giving them an understanding that the brain plays a significant role in pain perception, can reduce fear and anxiety associated with pain, potentially leading to better pain management outcomes.

Donald found this to be true when he learned about Dr. John Sarno's approach to pain. Through reading Sarno's *Healing Your Back*, Donald was able to feel the pain and then talk himself through it, reminding himself that the pain was not truly being created in his back, but instead it was coming from his brain. Over time, Donald linked his pain to the stress he experienced in his work and relationship. So, when he felt pain, he believed that this was his body protecting him from feeling his emotions tied to these stressful circumstances.

At these times, he would immediately do his diaphragmatic breathing exercises to stimulate his parasympathetic nervous system (PNS), a network of nerves that relaxes your body. He would then remind himself that the pain had nothing to do with his back and everything to do with his stress. For Donald, this process helped him significantly reduce his pain and often relieve it completely, likely due to the PNS's ability to settle our physiology and decrease hormones related to stress.

This process confirms that the way individuals think about and interpret their pain can significantly influence their experience and the connections that are made in the brain.

Improving Pain with Cognitive Behavioral Therapy

Donald was essentially rewiring his brain by using a few steps similar to those attending cognitive behavioral therapy sessions. I highly recommend exploring this process with a trained therapist, but you can start a few things on your own.

Cognitive behavioral therapies (CBT) suggest that repetitive negative thoughts and beliefs can exacerbate pain perception and contribute to chronic pain conditions. I hope this makes perfect sense now that you understand that science shows pain is produced in your brain 100 percent of the time.

Rewire the Brain to Eliminate Pain

To rewire your brain in order to reduce or eliminate pain, first you have to understand how you are reinforcing your experience of pain. Please remember that there is no judgment here. You are likely not aware of (and maybe do not yet believe) how a portion of the 6,000 to 70,000 thoughts you have per day could be reinforcing neural pathways in your brain related to pain.

> **Some scientists report that 90 to 95 percent of those thoughts are repetitive and out of our conscious awareness.**

Just like someone who has phantom limb pain isn't consciously choosing to have thoughts that create pain in their absent limb, you aren't choosing to reinforce neural networks that continue to contribute to your pain. But the fact remains that the pain is coming from your brain.

Similarly, if you have chronic pain for years (especially if the tangible and intangible triggers discussed in this book have been addressed) you are likely reinforcing thoughts, beliefs, and emotions about your pain without realizing it.

When I ask patients who are experiencing chronic pain these questions, their thoughts are nearly always focused on the anticipation of pain. They can see clearly how it will hurt and what they will have to do to compensate for the pain, and most can't imagine doing what they previously loved to do without pain. Those pain-related thought patterns have been reinforced over and over due to the vicious cycle of chronic pain.

It's a very easy trap to fall into, and you don't consciously choose it. It has nothing to do with weakness and everything to do with the neuroplasticity in your brain. Your body has been trying to protect you. You benefited from this protection at some point, but the protection you needed in the acute phase of pain is no longer as valuable to you now. You *can* keep yourself safe, move with little or no pain, and get back to doing many of the activities that you love. This is true even if you have arthritis, a pinched nerve, scar tissue, a failed surgery, bulging discs, or any tangible trigger from a blood test, MRI, or X-ray. Barring an emergent situation where your body needs immediate help, you can often overcome many physical findings present in previous test results and reduce or eliminate pain.

How to Stop Chronic Pain in its Tracks

First, you must realize what you are saying to yourself, what you are picturing in your mind, and even the emotions associated with these experiences in the past have reinforced the pain. Keep in mind that this isn't about ignoring thoughts, beliefs, or feelings regarding your pain. If that worked, you probably wouldn't have pain by now. You likely have been trying to ignore the pain and the feelings that go along with it for quite some time now. The key is becoming conscious of these thoughts, beliefs, or feelings, acknowledging them, learning from them, then letting them go and replacing them.

I know you might be thinking, "What? This is BS. I can't just think my pain away."

But neuroplasticity, a scientific truth about the brain, allows you to build your own constructive thoughts, beliefs, and feelings related to your past experience of pain and create a future that is pain-free, or at the very least, an existence with significantly less pain than you have now.

Still skeptical? Good, you should be! But I encourage you to remember what was discussed in Chapter 4 regarding placebo surgeries. Patients who thought they had a sham surgery on their knee for meniscus repair, on their disc for low back pain, or even on their brain for Parkinson's disease because they were put under anesthesia and their body was cut into, did better than those who had the actual surgical repair.

So, let's get to the how. Are you ready to do the work? I strongly encourage you to meet with a psychologist to help you through these steps, but here are some steps to begin if you feel comfortable starting while looking for a psychologist with whom to work.

And I can't help but think of this verse from the book *The Gospel of Thomas*. Though there are a few renditions of the quote, the one that has always resonated with me is verse 70:

> "If you bring forth what is within you, what you bring forth will save you. If you do not bring forth what is within you, what you do not bring forth will destroy you."

Let's get started.

Five Steps to Eliminate Pain From Your Brain and Body

In this section, there are five steps to help tap into your brain's neuroplasticity and begin the renovation process. Following these steps allows you to reconstruct and create new neural pathways that help you get rid of your pain, or at the very least, help you understand that it doesn't control you, you have the ability to influence it, and in time, as other patients have done, eliminate it.

Your five steps are:

1. **Find** the triggers
2. **Acknowledge** the triggers
3. **Learn** from them
4. **Reframe** and create new patterns
5. **Reinforce** these new patterns and pathways

Step 1: Find the Triggers

Sound familiar?

As discussed in previous chapters, triggers can be either tangible (observed or measured by you or someone else, e.g., a medical professional reading a blood test or physical therapist observing biomechanics) or intangible (difficult to measure and multifaceted, e.g., systemic inflammation, gut health, reinforced neural pathways).

The triggers I am referring to in this chapter are both tangible and intangible. But the difference is, you can observe the triggers yourself in order for you to get rid of them, instead of relying on someone else to point them out.

The process you are learning about here can move them from unconscious thoughts, feelings, and beliefs to your conscious awareness. In effect, you are moving them from intangible (not easily observed) to tangible (observed and at times, measurable).

WRITE IT DOWN

An effective way to accomplish this is by keeping a journal of how you are feeling when you have pain. Not the physical feeling, but the emotional feeling underneath it.

When you experience pain, stop and ask yourself: am I angry, sad, fearful or _____? You fill in the blank. Then record these thoughts and feelings related to the pain. These are an example of intangible triggers; however, as previously discussed, writing them down makes them tangible.

In the moment, if the pain is too distracting to answer that question, as close as you can to the painful event, ask yourself: what was I thinking and feeling right before this situation? You may identify a pattern of emotions or thoughts that are present which exacerbate the pain.

This is a common phenomenon related to those experiencing depression and anxiety. As discussed in Chapter 12, pain is increased in many people experiencing depression and anxiety.

USE VISUALIZATION

Another effective exercise to help you with journaling is to imagine yourself attempting to do something that in the past you enjoyed. What are the thoughts running through your head when you attempt to see yourself in the future doing something that was painful in the past? Simply write down any thoughts and feelings that come to you about the pain you experience. No judgment, just write it all down as if you were simply an observer watching the ticker tape of your thoughts roll through your brain.

Remember, if this exercise feels too confronting to you or you can't seem to bring anything up, seek out a psychologist to help you with this exercise.

CATASTROPHIZING

One thing this exercise can do is help you identify whether you are catastrophizing the pain you are experiencing.

Catastrophizing pain is one pattern that I see patients with chronic pain repeat. I see this often with chronic pelvic pain and chronic low back or neck pain, but catastrophizing is not limited to those areas.

Catastrophizing is a thought pattern in which individuals have magnified negative thoughts about their pain. Here are some examples:

Magnification: Thinking the pain will worsen uncontrollably.

- "My back pain is so bad today; it's only going to get worse."

Rumination: Focusing excessively on the pain and its impact.

- "I can't stop thinking about how much my knee hurts."

Helplessness: Believing there is nothing that can be done to alleviate the pain.

- "Nothing I do helps my pain. This is never going to go away."

Overgeneralization: Believing that because pain is present now, it will always be present.

THE BRAIN AND YOUR PAIN   319

- "My pain is bad today; it will always be this bad, and I'll never improve."

Catastrophic Predictions: Assuming the worst-case scenario will happen.

- "This pain means I'll end up in a wheelchair."

Catastrophizing can increase pain intensity and distress, reinforcing pain hypersensitivity and central sensitization, as we discussed earlier.

You can see the pattern of catastrophizing pain in Figures 13.2 and 13.3 from the medical journal *Neurology International*.

In Figure 13.2, you can see the pattern of catastrophizing due to fear of pain, and how this cycle reinforces more pain. Here is the pattern: Pain is experienced. You feel as though this pain will cause you harm. Fear

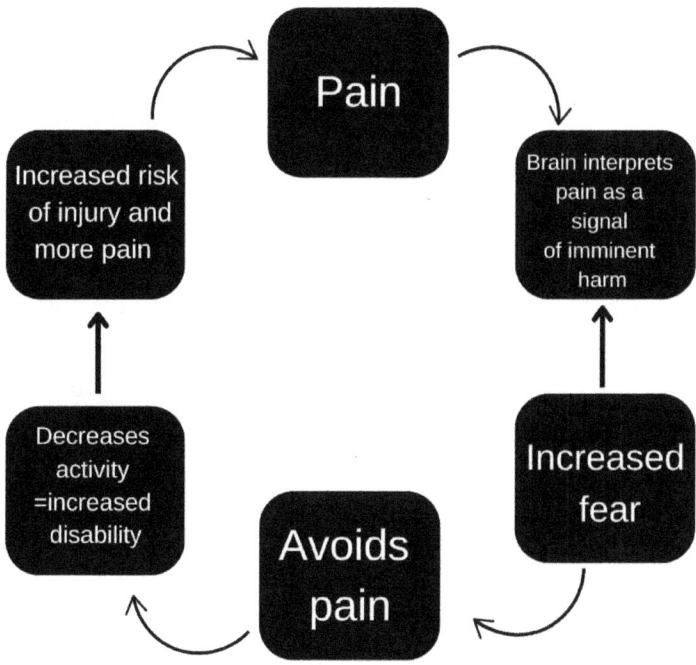

Figure 13.2 Catastrophizing

and anxiety increase. You avoid whatever you can to get away from the pain. You stop moving and exercising. You become weaker and increase risk of injury that can cause you pain. It's a vicious cycle.

Cognitive-Behavioral Therapy (CBT) is a powerful tool to address and change these destructive thought patterns. CBT works by helping individuals become aware of their negative thoughts, challenging these thoughts, and replacing them with more constructive and realistic ones. This process, known as cognitive restructuring, can significantly alleviate pain.

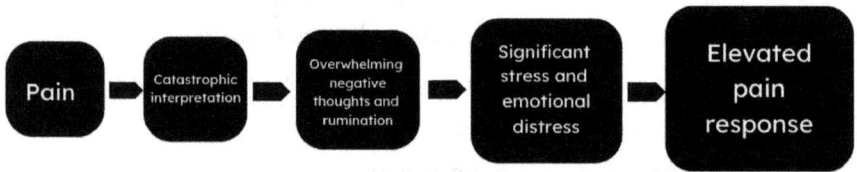

Figure 13.3

In Figure 13.3, you can see the pattern of increasing pain due to repeated overwhelming negative thoughts and rumination. You experience pain. You catastrophize the pain. Negative thoughts ensue and are repeated. This increases distress and contributes to pain increase.

Imagine Don, who is nearing retirement and loves playing golf and cycling with his son. What if, despite his active lifestyle, Don suffers from persistent low back pain that sometimes radiates down his leg? This pain, compounded by his worry about its impact on his hobbies and quality of life, leads to catastrophizing thoughts:

What if my pain never goes away?
What if I can't play golf anymore?
What if my son and I grow apart?

These thoughts not only increase his perception of pain, but also contribute to his overall distress.

Cognitive Behavioral Therapy would help him identify these negative thoughts. Don may be encouraged to keep a journal of his pain and associated thoughts, which will help him recognize patterns in his thinking. Once identified, it is possible to begin the process of cognitive restructuring. For instance, when Don thinks, *I'll never be able to run with my son again*, he instead can challenge this thought by asking, *What evidence do I have that I will never run again? What steps can I take to improve my chances of running again?* We will discuss this more later in Step Four: Reframe.

For now, let's start with step number one.

Step 1: Identify Triggers

Like Don did in his CBT sessions, you will likely see patterns within the information that you are writing down or recording during this experience. These patterns may consist of the same feelings or thoughts over and over. Some examples for you may be:

> I am sick and tired of this.
> Why me?
> Why does this keep happening to me?
> Why doesn't this go away? I have done everything I can.
> What is wrong with me?
> Why can't I find someone who can help me?
> I am afraid of_____.
> I am pissed off about _____.

Step 2: Acknowledge

You don't have to 'accept' what you wrote if you aren't ready to, or if you simply don't feel connected to the thoughts, beliefs, or feelings that appear. But they did come from you, so allow yourself to simply acknowledge that these thoughts came from your mind. No judgment. Realize that it is only information.

Acknowledgment may seem like a strange step, and it is one unfortunately many people skip only to have to come back to step two; acknowledge, to really move on.

Just think for a moment about the last time you were acknowledged for something, whether it was by another person who was important to you, or just by yourself.

Even though I may tell myself I don't need to be acknowledged by someone about something I did, it is still nice to hear. This acknowledgment oftentimes can soften resistance in our relationships with others, but in this case, acknowledgment may help lower our own inner resistance to working on and eventually reframing these thoughts, beliefs, and feelings.

Acknowledging what comes up can be as easy as repeating what you wrote to yourself and acknowledging that each statement came up for you, or simply acknowledging them as a whole. Writing a statement such as "I acknowledged the above," with your signature, is what some of my patients in the past have found helpful. But you do you. Everyone is different.

Now, a mini exercise within step two is to ask yourself: *when I think about these thoughts, beliefs, or feelings, does my pain change in any way?* This question and its answer may help you make a conscious connection as to whether these are the thoughts, feelings, or beliefs that will make a significant difference in the pain once they are reframed.

Step 3: Learn From the Triggers

Once you identify the patterns you are experiencing related to your thoughts, feelings, and beliefs around your pain, it's important to learn from them.

One of my patients, Evie, tried the exercise I recommended, and as she wrote down her statements and questions, she noticed something unsettling: her pain intensified. When we met again, she wasn't exactly thrilled with me. However, she admitted, "I did not realize how much these thoughts were actually contributing to my pain."

After she verbally acknowledged that these statements were what came up and it was just information to help her on her journey, we moved on to the next step, which was learning from them.

As Evie sat back in her seat, she pointed to her handwritten list and asked, "What on Earth can I possibly learn from that?"

Leaning forward in my chair, I peered at the upside down writing on the paper in front of me and gently pointed to an item on her list. "When you ask yourself, 'What can I learn from this?'" I said, my finger landing on a random entry, "like this one—'I am never going to get rid of this'—what comes up for you?"

Evie sighed, stared fiercely at me for a moment, and grabbed the glasses that rested on her chest, which were attached to a delicate strap around her neck. She placed them on her nose and peered down at the paper, then at me. "Honestly? The first thing that comes to mind is 'Absolutely nothing.' There's nothing I can learn from that," she said, leaning back and crossing her arms over her chest.

"Come on, Evie," I coaxed, "If you had to guess, what could you learn about yourself from that statement?"

I sat back in my chair, resting my index finger and thumb on my chin.

She sighed again, this time removing her glasses from the bridge of her nose and hugging her arms tightly over her chest. "I don't know," she muttered as she squirmed slightly in her seat, her eyes drifting away from mine. "Maybe . . ." she paused, her voice catching, "maybe it's more of a feeling than something I've learned. I guess it's . . ." Her eyes began to fill with tears, and I noticed a slight quiver in her chin as she looked down. "It's just that I feel so hopeless." As the words left her mouth, tears started to stream down her cheeks. "I'm sick and tired of feeling hopeless."

I reached out with a tissue, and she accepted it. And while her chest silently heaved up and down, Evie dabbed at the tears that had left moist trails on her face.

Evie wasn't someone who was used to feeling hopeless. She was a mother of three adult sons, whom she had raised on her own. Her tireless efforts had supported them all through college. Her resolve had always been strong. But the persistent pain in her feet and hip, which had plagued her for years and continued after surgery, kept her from the activities she loved and made her feel weak and feel like a failure. She felt as though her doctors did not believe her, especially after they assured her that her hip surgery had resolved all the structural issues. The final solution they offered was sending her to pain management, where, as she put it, "All they want to do is pump me full of different medications that I don't want to take."

I could feel Evie's frustration and despair emanating from her body. She had peeled away a protective layer she had built over the years that kept her vulnerability hidden from those around her, but more importantly from herself.

Cognitive restructuring turned out to be a welcome intervention for her. After six weekly sessions with myself and her cognitive behavioral therapist, she revealed to me that performing the journaling exercise was definitely uncomfortable at first, but the more she did it and applied what she learned, the less pain she experienced. She was also able to spend time with her only grandchild, which she said helped some joy return back into her life.

Dip Your Toe Into Cognitive Restructuring

Not ready to go to cognitive behavioral therapy, or maybe you have gone but haven't found a therapist yet that you connected with? Although working with a therapist is strongly recommended and significantly beneficial, you can still get started with step four in the process of tapping into your brain's neuroplasticity superpower by reframing the patterns you have identified in step one. If you get stuck on Step Three: Learning, let that go and move on to step four as this may help you move through the whole process. I do encourage you to go back to step three at some point.

Step 4: Reframe the Patterns

The American Psychological Association defines reframing as a "process of reconceptualizing a problem by seeing it from a different perspective. Altering the conceptual or emotional context of a problem often serves to alter perceptions of the problem's difficulty and to open up possibilities for solving it."

Now that you've identified thoughts that may be contributing to your pain—thoughts generated by the brain—and have acknowledged them, perhaps even gaining some valuable insights, let's begin the process of reframing. This can help you create those new neural pathways to reinforce in the next step and help you on your journey to a life where chronic pain no longer consumes you.

IN THE PAST, I USED TO . . .

In my clinic, I often ask my patients to use this phrase to begin the reframing process:

In the past, I used to _____ and now I choose to _____.

You will fill in the blanks with the thought you want to get rid of, and then put in the thought you would rather have. In other words, the first blank is for the potentially destructive thought of *my pain will never go away* that has been reinforced over and over based on your previous experiences.

You will then fill in the blank after 'and now I choose to', with how you want to see the situation instead. See the following example.

"In the past, I used to think that my pain will never go away. And now based on what I learned regarding the brain and how it changes with chronic pain, I choose to believe that I can improve it."

The second half of the response above is an example of 'dipping your toe' into the cognitive restructuring exercise. As you have read, 'I choose to believe that I can improve it' is not as strong of a statement as 'I choose to believe that I will never have pain for the rest of my life.' But the latter statement likely will not feel realistic.

I always encourage patients to begin with statements they can genuinely believe, rather than forcing strong affirmations that ignore their underlying thoughts, feelings, and beliefs. Starting with unrealistic statements, especially those that can never truly be accurate (since everyone experiences pain at times, and as discussed throughout this book, pain can be a valuable signal), risks not only failing to improve but potentially worsening the pain.

Through this process, you can, over time, replace negative thoughts with more constructive ones. This shift in thinking can reduce anxiety and significantly lower pain intensity.

CAN YOU REMEMBER A TIME WITHOUT PAIN?

Earlier in this chapter, I discussed imagining yourself doing something you used to love to do and writing down what you think and feel when this comes to mind. Can you see yourself participating in this activity without pain? Or better yet, can you see yourself participating in this activity pain-free, i.e. having fun, feeling joyful, moving freely?

If not, go back again to the time in your past when you could do the activity without pain, moving freely and enjoying it. What emotions were present? What thoughts are present when you think of that now?

You may find that when you recall these activities, you experience negative emotion. If you have negative emotions or thoughts, that is okay. Ask yourself: *where in my body do I feel this emotion or thought right now?* Write this down. Does your pain increase when you think about these times?

When I asked my patient Francis to do this exercise, here was her response:

"I hadn't thought about those days in a long time; you know, the days when I could just play with my grandkids, get down on the floor with them, laugh, and forget about everything else. It's funny, I never realized how much I took that for granted. Now, when I try to think about those moments, it's like they're behind a thick fog. I can see the edges of the memory, but it's hazy, distant, like a movie that's a little out of focus."

I asked Francis to picture spending time with her grandkids in the past. She closed her eyes and sat quietly for a moment as if she was traveling back in time in her mind's eye.

"What are you experiencing right now?" I asked

"I am trying to put myself back there." She wriggled in her seat and her hand moved to her lower back. "Wow, that's crazy. I can feel my low back stiffening right now, even though I know it did not hurt back then."

She opened her eyes and stood up from her seat with both hands on her low back as she walked away from my desk and back again. "That was so strange, like my brain couldn't connect to the version of me that was pain-free. I know, logically, that I did not have pain back then. I was active, I was present, and I enjoyed every moment. But when I close my eyes and try to imagine how that felt—how my body moved—it's like my mind can't access that memory. All I can feel is the pain I'm in right now."

The more we discussed what was happening in that moment—the emotions or thoughts —at first, the pain seemed to intensify. But once Francis identified the emotion attached to it, her pain began to subside.

It wasn't immediate. At first, the mention of her feelings seemed to amplify the pain. As we talked, Francis hesitated, her voice faltering as she started to acknowledge something deeper. Beneath the physical discomfort, there was an emotional layer she hadn't connected to her pain before. And then, as soon as she identified it—grief—the pieces began to fall into place. She described the feeling as a raw, aching sadness related to losing her husband, who had passed away two years earlier.

As she spoke about him, the tears flowed. After sharing a few memories of their life together, something unexpected happened. The tightness in her muscles started to release, the sharp edges of her pain dulled, and for the first time during our session, she took a deep, full breath. It was as if acknowledging the grief allowed the pain to soften its grip. The pain, which had felt so physical and immediate, wasn't gone completely, but it began to ease.

For Francis, this realization wasn't just about the connection between mind and body; it was a release. The grief she had been holding so tightly in her heart had found an outlet, and as it did, the physical pain that mirrored her emotional suffering began to lift.

Going forward from there, she was able to picture herself in the past moving freely without pain, and the next step was to work on seeing herself that way in the future.

FUTURE PACING

After our breakthrough moment discussing her grief, I asked Francis if she could do something different. I wanted her to picture herself in the future, moving freely without the burden of her chronic pain. At first, the concept of 'future pacing' seemed straightforward: if she could visualize a pain-free past, why not project that into her future? But as soon as I posed the question, her body language shifted again, her brow wrinkled as she tried to imagine a future event without pain.

"I don't know," she said after a long pause. "I can't really see it. It's like . . . it's not possible for me."

And just like it had before, her back stiffened. She could feel her body reacting to this request.

This struggle wasn't surprising. When someone has lived with pain for so long, the brain builds neural pathways that reinforce the experience. As Dr. Tara Swart, MD, PhD, explains in her book *The Source*, our brains don't just 'delete' old networks. Like data on a computer, remnants of these patterns stay on our mental hard drive, ready to resurface when triggered or reinforced. But, as Dr. Swart suggests, we can overwrite them by creating new neural connections. It takes time and repetition, but these new networks can become the new normal. Remember: neurons that fire together, wire together, according to neuropsychologist Donald Hebb. However, for Francis, those old networks—the ones tied to pain—were still dominant, making it difficult to envision a future where pain did not define her.

We worked on future pacing by repeating the first four previous steps:

1. Find the triggers (in Francis's case, grief was one of her triggers)
2. Acknowledge (as she acknowledged that grief from losing her husband was the cause of her pain, she was able to learn from it)

3. Learn (Francis realized she had to face the grief to help her let go of the pain)

4. Reframe (Seeing and experiencing her body moving freely in the past and future without pain)

To help Francis future pace, i.e. think of herself in the future without pain, we reviewed the reframing exercise.

I asked Francis to reframe what she previously thought about her pain by using the phrases listed at the beginning of step 4. As a reminder those were

In the past I used to _____

And now I choose to _____

Francis wrote: "In the past I used to see my pain as neverending and permanent. Now I choose to realize that the pain I had been experiencing was tied to the grief I have about my husband's passing. And though the grief may ebb and flow, I can let go of the physical pain and allow the memories of the good we had together prevail."

This exercise seemed to lift a heavy burden not just from her body but her heart.

Step 5: Reinforce

After Francis started to visualize herself at times doing simple, everyday activities—playing with her grandkids, taking a walk, bending down to tie her shoes—but without the pain, her face would contort slightly.

"I just don't see how I get there," she admitted. "It feels like it's too far away, like I'm fooling myself."

This was the mental block she had to break through. The reality was that her brain was wired to expect pain, and those expectations were shaping her mental imagery. What Francis was experiencing is exactly what research in neuroplasticity tells us: our beliefs, reinforced over time, create powerful neural networks that dictate how we perceive our reality.

Pain had become a constant part of her mental landscape, so imagining life without it felt foreign, even impossible.

We started small. Instead of asking Francis to see herself entirely pain-free, I asked her to picture a moment where her pain was just less noticeable—something manageable. This seemed more attainable for her, and as we practiced, she began to form a clearer picture of herself in the future. The image wasn't perfect, but it was a start.

Week by week, we built on this. Alongside her therapist, we used visualization exercises to help Francis 'see' herself living with less pain, even if the pain wasn't entirely gone. As she practiced visualizing the future without or with much less pain, when she felt resistance she would repeat her statements and fill in the blanks.

In the past I used to _____, and now I choose to _____. By doing this, Francis uncovered more beliefs she wanted to reframe. One in particular, "in the past I used to believe I would never get rid of this pain, and now I choose to believe I can get rid of the pain" was particularly powerful for her. Though we don't have imaging to see the changes, as her pain lessened, it was likely that her brain slowly began creating new connections. It wasn't an overnight change, but her persistence paid off. With each session, the resistance during her mental imagery began to fade. The future she couldn't previously envision started to come into focus.

"I'm not saying it's easy," she told me one day, "but now when I close my eyes, whether I think about moving without pain in the past or the future, I can actually see myself moving, doing things I like to do. It's not gone, but it's not in control anymore. It's just there, like background noise."

This shift was monumental for Francis. Over time, as she reframed her beliefs and her brain began reinforcing new, healthier patterns, her pain became more intermittent. The all-encompassing ache that once dominated her every movement and contributed to sleepless nights now had breaks; moments of relief. She wasn't as afraid to move, and she started to sleep without being awakened every few hours. And while the pain still returned, it wasn't as sharp, nor as constant. It became something she could manage.

But that wasn't the end of the story.

As part of her treatment plan, we reintroduced SoftWave therapy, the regenerative technology discussed in Chapter 7. After everything she had been through—the emotional breakthroughs, the cognitive reframing, and the steady work to reshape her neural pathways—SoftWave would now be more effective in addressing localized inflammation. Her response was almost immediate. Where the therapy had previously provided only very short-term relief, this time it worked in tandem with the mental shifts she had made.

Her body responded to the therapy in a profound way. The intermittent pain she had experienced during our work together began to diminish further, and the gaps between painful episodes grew longer.

"I can't believe how well this is working," Francis said during one of our last sessions. "I can finally picture my future self pain-free, something I did not even want to think about before. I'm living. And I never thought I'd say this, but I feel . . . hopeful."

For Francis, these five steps and SoftWave therapy marked the turning point in her journey. The pain she had experienced was no longer the defining factor in her life. With every step forward, she was creating a new normal—one where pain wasn't in control, and in her mind's eye, her future was bright, active, and full of promise.

Cognitive Restructuring to Reduce Pain

This process of cognitive restructuring that has been discussed in our five step formula isn't just for back pain. A comprehensive review in 2023 of fifteen different studies assessing the impact of cognitive behavioral therapy (CBT), the therapeutic technique related to cognitive restructuring, on chronic pain patients with knee and hip osteoarthritis showed promising results. CBT not only reduced pain but also improved sleep and overall quality of life. These findings underscore the potential of cognitive restructuring as an effective intervention for various types of chronic pain.

The key to its success lies in these techniques addressing both the conscious and unconscious thoughts and beliefs, essentially helping renovate and rewire the brain. By becoming aware of the destructive thoughts that occupy our mind and learning to replace them with constructive ones, we can begin to change the underlying cognitive patterns that contribute to chronic pain.

As you can see, the fifth step involves not just thinking differently, but to make a lasting change, it is important to continually **reinforce** what you created. After all, you wouldn't plant a seed but fail to water it daily if you want it to grow. When the plant is fully mature, it doesn't need your attention as often but does still need some care and adjustments from time to time to keep it alive and well.

The same is true for these new neural pathways that you are creating by tapping into the neuroplasticity in your brain to break the old pain cycle patterns. Over time, they will need to be reinforced and nurtured through repetition, stress management, and making healthy lifestyle choices discussed in the chapters of this book to optimize the health and resilience of your brain and body.

The following is a list of ways to reinforce steps one through four.

- **Repetition:** Repeating the steps for any new thoughts, beliefs, feelings, or emotions that present themselves. This process is truly like an onion; you will find there can be many layers under the one before it that will present keys to unlock and break the cycle of pain.

Evie and Francis found that keeping a journal on their phones helped to remind them about what unconscious thoughts had crept into her day that may not have been very supportive, not just related to pain but their overall well-being.

Reinforcing the changes in the thought patterns along with letting go of old beliefs and long-held emotions significantly impacted their results once we started back with SoftWave. Evie still wore her orthotics religiously, and they both kept up their exercises. They realized these commitments were the same as brushing their teeth each day. If they wanted an active life, they just had to do it. But in Evie's words, "Addressing my beliefs about pain was the key to my success."

- **Stress Management:** Engaging in activities that improve mood and reduce stress, such as visualization, mindfulness, meditation, and progressive muscle relaxation and activation.

For Don, stress management became a crucial part of his pain management strategy. By focusing on the present moment and practicing mindfulness, he noticed his stress levels drop, making the pain less and more manageable. Visualization techniques also played a key role in his recovery. He would imagine his back healing and see himself playing a pain-free round of golf or cycling with his son. Research shows that visualization reinforces not only brain patterns, but also physiological changes. A systematic review of mental imagery demonstrated that regularly visualizing strength training exercises can lead to muscle strength gains, even without physically performing the movements. While this doesn't replace the need for physical exercise, adding visualization can enhance the neuroplasticity of the brain and improve overall physical results.

More Evidence for Cognitive Behavior Therapy and Mindfulness in Pain

Research that evaluated over 300 individuals with low back pain were randomized to three groups.

Over 75 percent of participants reported at least one year of experiencing pain, and most reported pain on at least 160 of the previous 180 days. The average pain report was six out of ten, indicating moderate pain severity.

Participants were seen for in-group sessions for CBT or MBSR two hours a week for eight weeks maximum.

Group one received cognitive behavioral therapy (CBT) for a minimum of six sessions (max eight sessions).

Group two received instruction in mindfulness-based stress reduction techniques (MBSR) for two hours a week for eight weeks, plus a six-hour optional seminar.

Group three received the 'usual care,' i.e., whatever they wanted to pursue with the exception of CBT and MBSR.

Results:

Medications were used for pain at the beginning of the study by approximately 84 percent of the participants in the last week before starting.

Medication use at the end of fifty-two weeks was reduced for all groups

- Fifty-three percent of the participants in the 'usual care' group took medication a week prior to being asked.
- Forty-seven percent of the participants in the mindfulness group took medication for their back pain in the week prior to being asked.
- Forty-two percent of the participants in the CBT group took medication for their back pain in the week prior to being asked.

At fifty-two weeks, the percentage of participants that reported their pain "much better or completely gone" was as follows:

- Eighteen percent of the 'usual care' participants
- Thirty percent of the mindfulness group
- Thirty-two percent of the CBT group

Among adults with chronic pain, treatment with MBSR and CBT compared with usual care resulted in greater improvement in pain and fewer functional limitations at twenty-six weeks.

Understanding and altering the cognitive patterns that contribute to chronic pain helps lead to significant improvements in pain perception and quality of life. By incorporating strategies such as cognitive restructuring, mindfulness, and visualization, patients like you can find relief and regain control over their lives. This comprehensive approach highlights the importance of addressing the psychological aspects of pain, paving the way for more effective and lasting pain-management solutions.

- **Movement:** As discussed, a patient's hormone levels, gut health, and eating plan, as well as administering treatment modalities such as SoftWave to painful areas of the body, are essential for breaking free from pain. But many forget about how important movement is when we are reinforcing our cognitive approach to addressing chronic pain.

Most people realize that exercise is good for them. It helps us become stronger, more flexible, and more stable in our movements, helping to prevent injury. But when it comes to chronic pain, many people either intuitively or purposefully avoid movement as another protective mechanism. If they move too much, it hurts, so naturally, movement is often avoided.

But this avoidance and subsequent lack of movement results in:

- Biomechanical issues from weak, unstable, and tight muscles
- Less-than-optimal hormone levels
- Poor gut health
- Reinforcement of the fear-pain cycle

The more we repeat choosing inactivity to avoid pain and reinforce that pattern in our brain, the more we put ourselves at risk of injury and subsequently more pain. This inaction continues to reinforce neural networks in the brain related to avoiding activity and fear of more pain.

But a systematic review of ten research studies that investigated the effects of exercise on brain activity related to pain perception and quality of life revealed that exercise can potentially restore and even 'normalize' brain function in areas of the brain affected by chronic pain. The patients who demonstrated these changes in their brain typically reported improvements in pain and the quality of their life. The types of exercise most often included in the studies were Tai Chi, resistance training, or cardiovascular exercise.

For Don, once I personalized his exercise program, which included core stabilization and flexibility exercises to both take the stress off his back and improve the support of his lumbar spine, he was able to cycle and eventually run with his son without pain during and after. And both Evie and Francis were able to participate in their grandchildren's lives again.

Therefore, it can't be emphasized enough that movement must be a part of your Pain-Free Program to help you address pain that at one time was taking over your life. Find an experienced practitioner to help you find the right functional movement for your situation.

Not every person that I see needs to focus on tapping into the neuroplasticity of their brain to address pain. But adding these five steps into your pain-free program can only improve your results and help you live a happier, healthier life in the short and long run.

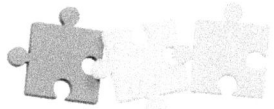

Key Pieces

Pain as a Brain-Centered Experience: Chronic pain can result from changes in the brain, not just the body. Understanding that pain is produced and regulated by the brain can shift how we approach pain management.

Pain Hypersensitivity and Central Sensitization: Chronic pain can lead to heightened sensitivity and hyperreaction to pain stimuli, a process driven by changes in the brain and nervous system.

Neuroplasticity's Role: The brain's ability to reorganize itself, known as neuroplasticity, can be harnessed to reduce chronic pain by creating new neural pathways and breaking old pain cycles.

Renovate and Rewire the Brain: There are five steps that can help patients with chronic pain tap into neuroplasticity:

1. Identify Triggers
2. Acknowledge
3. Learn
4. Reframe
5. Reinforce

Cognitive and Behavioral Interventions: Techniques like cognitive restructuring, mindfulness, and stress management can help retrain the brain's response to pain, significantly reducing pain intensity and improving quality of life.

Movement and Brain Changes: Incorporating personalized movement and exercise routines can help normalize brain function related to pain, supporting long-term pain management and recovery.

Want to dig a little bit deeper?
Check out our eBooks for Pain Free living at https://newyouhealthandwellness.com/ebooks

Afterword

As we conclude this journey toward understanding and managing pain, it's essential to reflect on the key strategies we've discussed. Joint and muscle pain is a multifaceted issue that requires a nuanced approach. Throughout this book, we've explored the limitations of conventional pain management—medications that can contribute to hypersensitivity, unnecessary surgeries, and injections like cortisone that may cause long-term harm.

Our exploration led us through a holistic approach to pain management and its elimination by addressing tangible triggers like biomechanics, muscle imbalances, and localized inflammation with manual therapy and effective modalities like SoftWave.

Additionally, we presented evidence supporting how intangible triggers related to gut health, food sensitivities, nutritional deficiencies, and hormonal imbalances could be contributing to persistent pain. By optimizing these areas, it's clear through our patient examples that these methods can reduce inflammation systemically and in the area being treated. This can result in the reduction or elimination of pain, as well as encouraging the body's own innate healing mechanisms to allow us to return to normal, pain-free activities.

We concluded with another trigger of persistent pain: the changes in the brain that develop over time and are related to chronic pain. We understand that these changes in the brain occur from the repetitive experience of pain, in addition to the neural networks formed from our thoughts, feelings, and beliefs about the pain experienced. Our journey led us to the power of neuroplasticity and how it can counteract pain hypersensitivity through cognitive restructuring. This includes cognitive-behavioral therapy (CBT) and other methods that address thought patterns such as catastrophizing. By identifying and challenging these thoughts, individuals can significantly alter their pain experience and reduce distress.

Mindfulness, meditation, visualization, and appropriate exercise provide powerful tools for pain management. These practices reduce pain perception and enhance emotional well-being and resilience. Incorporating these techniques into daily life can help individuals cope with, alleviate, and even eliminate chronic pain.

In closing, the journey toward pain-free living involves continuous learning, adaptation, and perseverance. The strategies and insights provided here are meant to empower you to take control of your pain and improve your quality of life. Embrace the tools and knowledge you've gained and apply them with confidence and compassion for yourself. Reach out for support when needed and believe in your capacity for healing and resilience. Your journey is unique, and with each step you are moving closer to a life less burdened by pain.

Thank you for joining me on this journey. Here's to a future where you can enjoy your activities, connect deeply with your loved ones by sharing in activities, and live each day to the fullest, free from chronic pain.

Authors Note: Not Sure Which Puzzle Pieces Are the Most Important Pieces for You?

Here's what to do next...

Some readers who have finished *The Pain Free Formula* have asked, "Where do I go from here?" With so many potential factors contributing to pain—biomechanics, hormones, food sensitivities, gut health, or the emotional aspect of dealing with chronic pain—it can feel overwhelming to know where to start.

To help you narrow down the areas most relevant to your situation, I've created a free quiz designed to guide you in identifying key contributors to your pain. Once completed, you'll receive a personalized report that can help you, your healthcare provider, or our team target the root causes of your pain.

If you choose to pursue services with us or another practitioner, this report will serve as a valuable tool, offering insight into the areas that may require attention to help you finally achieve lasting relief.

To take the quiz, visit:
https://newyouhealthandwellness.com/the-pain-free-formula-quiz

Warmly,

Stacey Roberts

OTHER RESOURCES:

Check out The Pain-Free Podcast at www.thepainfreepodcast.com Go to https://newyouhealthandwellness.com/ebooks to find out more about how you can get rid of muscle and joint pain. These short-form eBooks are workbooks with simple steps to follow to dig deeper into each of the areas discussed in The Pain Free Formula.

Sources

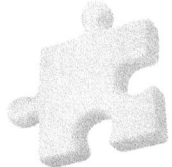

Chapter 1: Unmasking Your Pain
Keller, H. (1903). Optimism, An Essay, by Helen Keller.

Orthopedic Braces And Supports Market Size, Share & Trends Analysis Report By Product (Braces & Supports Type, Pain Management Products), By End-use (Orthopedic Clinics, OTC), By Region, And Segment Forecasts, 2024—2030. (n.d.). https://www.grandviewresearch.com/industry-analysis/orthopedic-braces-support-systems-market

Research, P. (2024, June 3). *Pain Management Drugs Market Size To Hit USD 120.16 Bn By 2033.* https://www.precedenceresearch.com/pain-management-drugs-market

Chapter 2: Wired for Warning: How Pain Works
Nagasako, E. M., Oaklander, A. L., & Dworkin, R. H. (2003). Congenital insensitivity to pain: an update. *Pain, 101*(3), 213–219. https://doi.org/10.1016/S0304-3959(02)00482-7

"Ouch, that hurts!" The science of pain | NIH MedlinePlus Magazine. (n.d.). NIH MedlinePlus Magazine. https://magazine.medlineplus.gov/article/ouch-that-hurts-the-science-of-pain

Attia, P., & Attia, P. (2024, February 7). *#287 - Lower back pain: causes, treatment, and prevention of lower back injuries and pain | Stuart McGill,. . .* Peter Attia. https://peterattiamd.com/stuartmcgill/

Chapter 3: Chronic Pain
Kindle, P. A., & Delavega, E. (2018). Originals: How non-conformists move the world. By Adam Grant, New York, NY: Viking Press, 2016, 322 pages. ISBN: 978-0-525-42956-2. Journal of Human Behavior in the Social Environment, 28(5), 673–675. https://doi.org/10.1080/10911359.2018.1449694

Donohue J. (2006). A history of drug advertising: the evolving roles of consumers and consumer protection. *The Milbank quarterly*, 84(4), 659–699. https://doi.org/10.1111/j.1468-0009.2006.00464.x

Spending on Consumer Advertising for Top-Selling Prescription Drugs in U.S. Favors Those With Low Added Benefit. (2023, February 22). *Johns Hopkins Bloomberg School of Public Health*. https://publichealth.jhu.edu/2023/spending-on-consumer-advertising-for-top-selling-prescription-drugs-in-us-favors-those-with-low-added-benefit Healthcare & pharmaceutical industry digital ad spend in the U.S. *2011-2024*. (2023, October 11).

Statista.https://www.statista.com/statistics/235966/us-healthcare-and-pharmaceutical-industry-online-ad-spending/

Non-Steroidal Anti-Inflammatory Drugs Market Skyrockets: Witness Impressive US$ 28.7 billion by 2030 and Striking CAGR of 6.0%—By PMI. (2023, November 9). *GlobeNewswire News Room*. https://www.globenewswire.com/en/news-release/2023/11/09/2777358/0/en/Non-Steroidal-Anti-Inflammatory-Drugs-Market-Skyrockets-Witness-Impressive-US-28-7-billion-by-2030-and-Striking-CAGR-of-6-0-By-PMI.html

Parisien, M., Lima, L. V., Dagostino, C., El-Hachem, N., Drury, G. L., Grant, A. V., Huising, J., Verma, V., Meloto, C. B., Silva, J. R., Dutra, G. G. S., Markova, T., Dang, H., Tessier, P. A., Slade, G. D., Nackley, A. G., Ghasemlou, N., Mogil, J. S., Allegri, M., & Diatchenko, L. (2022). Acute inflammatory response via neutrophil activation protects against the development of chronic pain. *Science Translational Medicine*, 14(644), eabj9954. https://doi.org/10.1126/scitranslmed.abj9954

Wang, B., Wu, L., Chen, J. *et al.* Metabolism pathways of arachidonic acids: mechanisms and potential therapeutic targets. *Sig Transduct Target Ther* 6, 94 (2021). https://doi.org/10.1038/s41392-020-00443-w

Kaeley, G. S., Thway, M., & Dodani, S. Injectable Corticosteroid Use in Musculoskeletal Care Specialties [abstract]. *Arthritis Rheumatol*. 2016; 68 (suppl 10). https://acrabstracts.org/abstract/injectable-corticosteroid-use-in-musculoskeletal-care-specialties/ Professional, C. C. M. (2024, May 1). *NSAIDs (Nonsteroidal Anti-Inflammatory Drugs)*. Cleveland Clinic.https://my.clevelandclinic.org/health/treatments/11086-non-steroidal-anti-inflammatory-medicines-nsaids

BioSpace. (2022, July 14). *Non-steroidal Anti-inflammatory Drugs Market Size USD 31.45 Billion by 2030.* https://www.biospace.com/article/non-steroidal-anti-inflammatory-drugs-market-size-usd-31-45-billion-by-2030

Ayoub, S. S. (2021). Paracetamol (acetaminophen): A familiar drug with an unexplained mechanism of action. *Temperature* (Austin, Tex.), 8(4), 351–371. https://doi.org/10.1080/23328940.2021.1886392

Leopoldino AO, Machado GC, Ferreira PH, et al. Paracetamol versus placebo for knee and hip osteoarthritis. *Cochrane Database Syst Rev.* 2019(2):CD013273
MacIntyre, I. M., Turtle, E. J., Farrah, T. E., Graham, C., Dear, J. W., Webb, D. J., & PATH-BP (Paracetamol in Hypertension–Blood Pressure) Investigators* (2022). Regular Acetaminophen Use and Blood Pressure in People With Hypertension: The PATH-BP Trial. *Circulation,* 145(6), 416–423. https://doi.org/10.1161/CIRCULATIONAHA.121.056

Conaghan, P. G., Arden, N., Avouac, B., Migliore, A., & Rizzoli, R. (2019). Safety of Paracetamol in Osteoarthritis: What Does the Literature Say?. *Drugs & Aging,* 36(Suppl. 1), 7–14. https://doi.org/10.1007/s40266-019-00658-9

Lee W. M. (2017). Acetaminophen (APAP) hepatotoxicity-Isn't it time for APAP to go away?. *Journal of hepatology,* 67(6), 1324–1331. https://doi.org/10.1016/j.jhep.2017.07.005
Are Your Painkillers Actually Killing You? (2006, December 22). ABC News. https://abcnews.go.com/Health/PainManagement/story?id=2739177&page=1
Acetaminophen (Oral Route, Rectal Route). (2024, March 5). https://www.mayoclinic.org/drugs-supplements/acetaminophen-oral-route-rectal-route/side-effects/drg-20068480

Benyamin, R., Trescot, A. M., Datta, S., Buenaventura, R., Adlaka, R., Sehgal, N., Glaser, S. E., & Vallejo, R. (2008). Opioid complications and side effects. *Pain Physician,* 11(2 Suppl), S105–S120.

Klenø, A. N., Sørensen, H. T., & Pedersen, A. B. (2022). Time trends in use of non-steroidal anti-inflammatory drugs and opioids one year after total hip arthroplasty due to osteoarthritis during 1996-2018: a population-based cohort study of 103,209 patients. *Osteoarthritis and Cartilage,* 30(10), 1376–1384.

Faaem, S. W. M. M. F. (2021, July 29). *Right-sizing opioid prescriptions after surgery*. Harvard Health. https://www.health.harvard.edu/blog/right-sizing-opioid-prescriptions-after-surgery-202107292557

FDA.gov. (2018, February 5). Understanding Unapproved Use of Approved Drugs "Off Label." *FDA.gov*. Retrieved September 2, 2024, from https://www.fda.gov/patients/learn-about-expanded-access-and-other-treatment-options/understanding-unapproved-use-approved-drugs-label

Van Norman, G. A. (2023). Off-Label Use vs Off-Label Marketing of Drugs: Part 1: Off-Label Use-Patient Harms and Prescriber Responsibilities. *JACC. Basic to Translational Science*, 8(2), 224–233. https://doi.org/10.1016/j.jacbts.2022.12.011

Off-Label Drugs: What You Need to Know | Agency for Healthcare Research and Quality. (n.d.-b). https://www.ahrq.gov/patients-consumers/patient-involvement/off-label-drug-usage.html

Peter Yi, Peter Pryzbylkowski, Opioid Induced Hyperalgesia, *Pain Medicine*, Volume 16, Issue suppl_1, October 2015, Pages S32–S36, https://doi.org/10.1111/pme.12914
Yasaei, R., Katta, S., Patel, P., & Saadabadi, A. (2024, February 21). *Gabapentin*. StatPearls—NCBI Bookshelf. https://www.ncbi.nlm.nih.gov/books/NBK493228/
Gabapentin (Oral Route). (2024, August 7). https://www.mayoclinic.org/drugs-supplements/Gabapentin-oral-route/side-effects/drg-20064011

FDA Warns About Serious Breathing Problems with seizure and nerve pain medications Gabapentin. (2022, January 19). *FDA.gov*. https://www.fda.gov/drugs/fda-drug-safety-podcasts/fda-warns-about-serious-breathing-problems-seizure-and-nerve-pain-medicines-Gabapentin-neurontin

Mattson, C. L., Chowdhury, F., & Gilson, T. P. (2022). Notes from the Field: Trends in Gabapentin Detection and Involvement in Drug Overdose Deaths — 23 States and the District of Columbia, 2019–2020. *MMWR Morbidity and Mortality Weekly Report*, 71(19), 664–666. https://doi.org/10.15585/mmwr.mm7119a3

Anderson, D. B., & Shaheed, C. A. (2022). Medications for Treating Low Back Pain in Adults. Evidence for the Use of Paracetamol, Opioids, Nonsteroidal Anti-inflammatories, Muscle Relaxants, Antibiotics, and Antidepressants: An Overview for

Musculoskeletal Clinicians. *The Journal of orthopaedic and sports physical therapy*, 52(7), 425–431. https://doi.org/10.2519/jospt.2022.10788

Professional, C. C. M. (2024c, August 2). *Muscle Relaxers*. Cleveland Clinic. https://my.clevelandclinic.org/health/treatments/24686-muscle-relaxers

Alvarez, C. A., Mortensen, E. M., Makris, U. E., Berlowitz, D. R., Copeland, L. A., Good, C. B., Amuan, M. E., & Pugh, M. J. (2015). Association of skeletal muscle relaxers and antihistamines on mortality, hospitalizations, and emergency department visits in elderly patients: a nationwide retrospective cohort study. *BMC geriatrics*, 15, 2. https://doi.org/10.1186/1471-2318-15-2

Penn Medicine. (2020, June 25). Long-term Use of Muscle Relaxants Has Skyrocketed Since 2005. *www.pennmedicine.org*. Retrieved September 2, 2023, from https://www.pennmedicine.org/news/news-releases/2020/june/long-term-use-of-muscle-relaxants-has-skyrocketed-since-2005

Professional, C. C. M. (2024b, August 2). *Muscle Relaxers*. Cleveland Clinic. https://my.clevelandclinic.org/health/treatments/24686-muscle-relaxers

Lin, C. Y., Huang, S. C., Tzou, S. J., Yin, C. H., Chen, J. S., Chen, Y. S., & Chang, S. T. (2022). A Positive Correlation between Steroid Injections and Cuff Tendon Tears: A Cohort Study Using a Clinical Database. *International journal of environmental research and public health*, 19(8), 4520. https://doi.org/10.3390/ijerph19084520

Thomas, K., & Schonmann, Y. (2021). Orthopaedic corticosteroid injections and risk of acute coronary syndrome: a cohort study. *The British journal of general practice : the journal of the Royal College of General Practitioners*, 71(703), e128–e133. https://doi.org/10.3399/bjgp20X713945

Kompel, A. J., Roemer, F. W., Murakami, A. M., Diaz, L. E., Crema, M. D., & Guermazi, A. (2019). Intra-articular corticosteroid injections in the hip and knee: Perhaps not as safe as we thought? *Radiology*, 293(3), 656–663. https://doi.org/10.1148/radiol.2019190341

Grey, H. (2019, October 15). Steroid Injections in the Knee and Hip Can Cause More Damage Than Previously Realized. *Healthline*. https://www.healthline.com/health-news/steroid-injections-in-the-knee-and-hip-can-cause-more-damag

Liu, S. H., Dubé, C. E., Eaton, C. B., Driban, J. B., McAlindon, T. E., & Lapane, K. L. (2018). Long-Term Effectiveness of Intra-Articular Injections on Patient-Reported Symptoms in Knee Osteoarthritis. *The Journal of Rheumatology*, 45(9), 1316–1324. https://doi.org/10.3899/jrheum.171385

Xiong, Y., Gong, C., Peng, X., Liu, X., Su, X., Tao, X., Li, Y., Wen, Y., & Li, W. (2023). Efficacy and safety of platelet-rich plasma injections for the treatment of osteoarthritis: a systematic review and meta-analysis of randomized controlled trials. *Frontiers in Medicine*, 10, 1204144. https://doi.org/10.3389/fmed.2023.1204144

Maleitzke, T., Elazaly, H., Festbaum, C., Eder, C., Karczewski, D., Perka, C., Duda, G. N., & Winkler, T. (2020). Mesenchymal Stromal Cell-Based Therapy-An Alternative to Arthroplasty for the Treatment of Osteoarthritis? A State of the Art Review of Clinical Trials. *Journal of Clinical Medicine*, 9(7), 2062. https://doi.org/10.3390/jcm9072062
Pozek, J. P., Beausang, D., Baratta, J. L., & Viscusi, E. R. (2016). The Acute to Chronic Pain Transition: Can Chronic Pain Be Prevented?. *The Medical Clinics of North America*, 100(1), 17–30. https://doi.org/10.1016/j.mcna.2015.08.005

Thapa, P., & Euasobhon, P. (2018). Chronic postsurgical pain: current evidence for prevention and management. *The Korean Journal of Pain*, 31(3), 155–173. https://doi.org/10.3344/kjp.2018.31.3.155

Kuo SJ, Su YH, Hsu SC, Huang PH, Hsia CC, Liao CY, Chen SH, Wu RW, Hsu CC, Lai YC, Liu DY, Ku NE, Chen JF, Ko JY. Effects of Adding Extracorporeal Shockwave Therapy (ESWT) to Platelet-Rich Plasma (PRP) among Patients with Rotator Cuff Partial Tear: A Prospective Randomized Comparative Study. J Pers Med. 2024 Jan 10;14(1):83. doi: 10.3390/jpm14010083. PMID: 38248784; PMCID: PMC10820784.
Liu SC, Qiao XF, Tang QX, Li XG, Yang JH, Wang TQ, Xiao YJ, Qiao JM. Therapeutic efficacy of extracorporeal shock wave combined with hyaluronic acid on knee osteoarthritis. Medicine (Baltimore). 2019 Feb;98(8):e14589. doi: 10.1097/MD.0000000000014589. PMID: 30813181; PMCID: PMC6408132.

Hsu CC, Cheng JH, Wang CJ, Ko JY, Hsu SL, Hsu TC. Shockwave Therapy Combined with Autologous Adipose-Derived Mesenchymal Stem Cells Is Better than with Human Umbilical Cord Wharton's Jelly-Derived Mesenchymal Stem Cells on Knee Osteoarthritis. Int J Mol Sci. 2020 Feb 12;21(4):1217. doi: 10.3390/ijms21041217. PMID: 32059379; PMCID: PMC7072878.

Cheng JH, Yen KT, Chou WY, Jhan SW, Hsu SL, Ko JY, Wang CJ, Kuo CA, Wu SY, Hsu TC, Hsu CC. Autologous Adipose-Derived Mesenchymal Stem Cells Combined with Shockwave Therapy Synergistically Ameliorates the Osteoarthritic Pathological Factors in Knee Joint. Pharmaceuticals (Basel). 2021 Apr 1;14(4):318. doi: 10.3390/ph14040318. PMID: 33916108; PMCID: PMC8065528.

Chapter 4: Surgical Shadows: Understand the Risks and Limitations of Surgery
Turner, T. (2018, April 17). JAMA: Unnecessary Joint Replacements Cost Americans $8.3 Billion. *Drugwatch.com*. https://www.drugwatch.com/news/2018/03/19/jama-unnecessary-joint-replacements-cost-americans-8-3-billion/

Stone, K. (2019, July 19). *Why most total knee replacements are not needed*. San Francisco Examiner. https://www.sfexaminer.com/lifestyles/why-most-total-knee-replacements-are-not-needed/article_2bbb3cbe-5e64-5f6d-90c0-fae32e1985d7.html

Greengard, S. (2020, March 31). *All You Want to Know About Total Knee Replacement*. Healthline. https://www.healthline.com/health-news/one-third-knee-replacements-unnecessary-070114

Valtetsiotis, K., Di Martino, A., Brunello, M., Tassinari, L., D'Agostino, C., Traina, F., & Faldini, C. (2023). The Potential Role of Gut Bacteriome Dysbiosis as a Leading Cause of Periprosthetic Infection: A Comprehensive Literature Review. *Microorganisms*, *11*(7), 1778. https://doi.org/10.3390/microorganisms11071778

Riddle, D. L., Jiranek, W. A., & Hayes, C. W. (2014). Use of a validated algorithm to judge the appropriateness of total knee arthroplasty in the United States: a multicenter longitudinal cohort study. *Arthritis & rheumatology (Hoboken, N.J.)*, *66*(8), 2134–2143. https://doi.org/10.1002/art.38685

Lam V, Teutsch S, Fielding J. Hip and Knee Replacements: A Neglected Potential Savings Opportunity. *JAMA*. 2018;319(10):977–978. doi:10.1001/jama.2018.2310

Stone, K. R. (2023, January 12). *Avoiding Total Knee Replacements*. https://www.stoneclinic.com/blog/avoiding-total-knee-replacements

Matar, H. E., Porter, P. J., & Porter, M. L. (2021). Metal allergy in primary and revision total knee arthroplasty : a scoping review and evidence-based practical approach. *Bone &*

joint open, 2(10), 785–795. https://doi.org/10.1302/2633-1462.210.BJO-2021-0098.R1

Oltean-Dan, D., Apostu, D., Tomoaia, G., Kerekes, K., Păiuşan, M. G., Bardas, C. A., & Benea, H. R. C. (2022). Causes of revision after total hip arthroplasty in an orthopedics and traumatology regional center. *Medicine and Pharmacy Reports*, 95(2), 179–184. https://doi.org/10.15386/mpr-2136

Schwartz, A. M., Farley, K. X., Guild, G. N., & Bradbury, T. L., Jr. (2020). Projections and Epidemiology of Revision Hip and Knee Arthroplasty in the United States to 2030. *The Journal of Arthroplasty*, 35(6S), S79–S85. https://doi.org/10.1016/j.arth.2020.02.030

Van der Merwe, J. M. (2021). Metal Hypersensitivity in Joint Arthroplasty. *Journal of the American Academy of Orthopaedic Surgeons. Global research & reviews*, 5(3), e20.00200. https://doi.org/10.5435/JAAOSGlobal-D-20-00200et

Mahdi, A., Svantesson, M., Wretenberg, P., & Hälleberg-Nyman, M. (2020). Patients' experiences of discontentment one year after total knee arthroplasty- a qualitative study. *BMC Musculoskeletal Disorders*, 21(1), 29. https://doi.org/10.1186/s12891-020-3041-y

Hafkamp, F. J., Gosens, T., de Vries, J., & den Oudsten, B. L. (2020). Do dissatisfied patients have unrealistic expectations? A systematic review and best-evidence synthesis in knee and hip arthroplasty patients. *EFORT open reviews*, 5(4), 226–240. https://doi.org/10.1302/2058-5241.5.190015

Kurtz, S., Ong, K., Lau, E., Mowat, F., & Halpern, M. (2007). Projections of primary and revision hip and knee arthroplasty in the United States from 2005 to 2030. *The Journal of bone and joint surgery. American volume*, 89(4), 780–785. https://doi.org/10.2106/JBJS.F.00222

Neuprez, A., Neuprez, A. H., Kaux, J. F., Kurth, W., Daniel, C., Thirion, T., Huskin, J. P., Gillet, P., Bruyère, O., & Reginster, J. Y. (2020). Total joint replacement improves pain, functional quality of life, and health utilities in patients with late-stage knee and hip osteoarthritis for up to 5 years. *Clinical Rheumatology*, 39(3), 861–871. https://doi.org/10.1007/s10067-019-04811-y

Alshammari, H. S., Alshammari, A. S., Alshammari, S. A., & Ahamed, S. S. (2023). Prevalence of Chronic Pain After Spinal Surgery: A Systematic Review and

Meta-Analysis. *Cureus, 15*(7), e41841. https://doi.org/10.7759/cureus.41841

Cram, P., Landon, B. E., Matelski, J., Ling, V., Perruccio, A. V., Paterson, J. M., & Rampersaud, Y. R. (2019). Utilization and Outcomes for Spine Surgery in the United States and Canada. *Spine, 44*(19), 1371–1380. https://doi.org/10.1097/BRS.0000000000003083

Research, I. (2023, October 5). *How Many Spinal Fusions are Performed Each Year in the United States?* iData Research. https://idataresearch.com/how-many-instrumented-spinal-fusions-are-performed-each-year-in-the-united-states

Parker, S. L., Mendenhall, S. K., Godil, S. S., Sivasubramanian, P., Cahill, K., Ziewacz, J., & McGirt, M. J. (2015). Incidence of Low Back Pain After Lumbar Discectomy for Herniated Disc and Its Effect on Patient-reported Outcomes. *Clinical orthopaedics and related research, 473*(6), 1988–1999. https://doi.org/10.1007/s11999-015-4193-1

Tonosu, J., Oka, H., Higashikawa, A., Okazaki, H., Tanaka, S., & Matsudaira, K. (2017). The associations between magnetic resonance imaging findings and low back pain: A 10-year longitudinal analysis. *PloS one, 12*(11), e0188057. https://doi.org/10.1371/journal.pone.0188057

Jensen, M. C., Brant-Zawadzki, M. N., Obuchowski, N., Modic, M. T., Malkasian, D., & Ross, J. S. (1994). Magnetic Resonance Imaging of the Lumbar Spine in People without Back Pain. *New England Journal of Medicine, 331*(2), 69–73. https://doi.org/10.1056/nejm199407143310201

Brinjikji, W., Luetmer, P. H., Comstock, B., Bresnahan, B. W., Chen, L. E., Deyo, R. A., Halabi, S., Turner, J. A., Avins, A. L., James, K., Wald, J. T., Kallmes, D. F., & Jarvik, J. G. (2015). Systematic literature review of imaging features of spinal degeneration in asymptomatic populations. *AJNR. American journal of neuroradiology, 36*(4), 811–816. https://doi.org/10.3174/ajnr.A4173

Jonas WB, Crawford C, Colloca L, Kaptchuk TJ, Moseley B, Miller FG, Kriston L, Linde K, Meissner K. To what extent are surgery and invasive procedures effective beyond a placebo response? A systematic review with meta-analysis of randomized, sham controlled trials. BMJ Open. 2015 Dec 11;5(12):e009655. doi: 10.1136/bmjopen-2015-009655. PMID: 26656986; PMCID: PMC4679929.

Tran, A. A., & Prasad, V. (2023). Visualizing the randomized sham-controlled trial in orthopedic research: proposed steps to conducting a total knee arthroplasty randomized controlled trial. *Journal of Comparative Effectiveness Research, 12*(3). https://doi.org/10.57264/cer-2021-0275

2.5 million Americans living with artificial hip, 4.7 million with artificial knee. (2014, March 14). ScienceDaily. https://www.sciencedaily.com/releases/2014/03/140314093737.htm

SchrÃ¸der CP, Skare Ã˜, ReikerÃ¥s O, *et al*Sham surgery versus labral repair or biceps tenodesis for type II SLAP lesions of the shoulder: a three-armed randomized clinical trial *British Journal of Sports Medicine* 2017;**51**:1759-1766.

Khan M, Alolabi B, Horner N, Bedi A, Ayeni OR, Bhandari M. Surgery for shoulder impingement: a systematic review and meta-analysis of controlled clinical trials. CMAJ Open. 2019 Mar 7;7(1):E149-E158. doi: 10.9778/cmajo.20180179. PMID: 30846616; PMCID: PMC6411477.

How do exercise and arthritis fit together? (n.d.). Mayo Clinic. https://www.mayoclinic.org/diseases-conditions/arthritis/in-depth/arthritis/art-20047971#

Chapter 5: Why Won't My Pain Go Away
Fariduddin MM, Bansal N. Hypothyroid Myopathy. [Updated 2022 Aug 8]. In: StatPearls [Internet]. Treasure Island (FL): StatPearls Publishing; 2023 Jan-. Available from: https://www.ncbi.nlm.nih.gov/books/NBK519513/

Klyne, D. M., Barbe, M. F., James, G., & Hodges, P. W. (2021). Does the Interaction between Local and Systemic Inflammation Provide a Link from Psychology and Lifestyle to Tissue Health in Musculoskeletal Conditions?. *International Journal of Molecular Sciences, 22*(14), 7299. https://doi.org/10.3390/ijms22147299

Caio, G., Volta, U., Sapone, A., Leffler, D. A., De Giorgio, R., Catassi, C., & Fasano, A. (2019). Celiac disease: a comprehensive current review. *BMC medicine, 17*(1), 142. https://doi.org/10.1186/s12916-019-1380-z

Priyadarshini, S., Asghar, A., Shabih, S., & Kasireddy, V. (2022). Celiac Disease Masquerading as Arthralgia. *Cureus, 14*(6), e26387. https://doi.org/10.7759/cureus.26387

Ghoneim, Sara MD1; Dalal, Shaman MD1; Shah, Aun R. MD, MRCP2; Hamid, Osama MD, MRCPI3; Dhorepatil, Aneesh MD1; Ali, Rubab MBBS4; Arshad, Muhammad Arsalan MD5; Chandan, Saurabh MD6. S1283 The Epidemiology of Celiac Disease Among Adult Patients: A Population-Based Study. The American Journal of Gastroenterology 115():p S644-S645, October 2020. | DOI: 10.14309/01. ajg.0000707180.15506.d7

Lin, H. M., Hsieh, P. S., Chen, N. C., Tsai, C. H., Kuo, W. F., Lee, Y. L., & Hung, K. C. (2023). Impact of cognitive behavior therapy on osteoarthritis-associated pain, insomnia, depression, fatigue, and physical function in patients with knee/hip osteoarthritis: A systematic review and meta-analysis of randomized controlled trials. *Frontiers in medicine*, *9*, 1083095. https://doi.org/10.3389/fmed.2022.1083095

Chapter 6: Biomechanics and Insufficient Movement Patterns: A Common Tangible Trigger
National Research Council (US) and Institute of Medicine (US) Panel on Musculoskeletal Disorders and the Workplace. Musculoskeletal Disorders and the Workplace: Low Back and Upper Extremities. Washington (DC): National Academies Press (US); 2001. 6, Biomechanics. Available from: https://www.ncbi.nlm.nih.gov/books/NBK222434/

Chapter 7: Shockwave: The Most Effective Modality to Get Rid of Localized Pain
Wu, S. S., Ericson, K. J., & Shoskes, D. A. (2020). Retrospective comparison of focused shockwave therapy and radial wave therapy for men with erectile dysfunction. *Translational andrology and urology*, *9*(5), 2122–2128. https://doi.org/10.21037/tau-20-911

Physical principles of ESWT | ISMST. (n.d.-b). https://shockwavetherapy.org/physical-principles-of-eswt/

Chapter 8: Tackling the Intangible Triggers
Keller, H. (2016). The Story of My Life. Om Books International.
Meints, S. M., & Edwards, R. R. (2018). Evaluating psychosocial contributions to chronic pain outcomes. *Progress in neuro-psychopharmacology & biological psychiatry*, *87*(Pt B), 168–182. https://doi.org/10.1016/j.pnpbp.2018.01.017

Chapter 9: Gut Health and Joint Pain
Romero-Figueroa, M. D. S., Ramírez-Durán, N., Montiel-Jarquín, A. J., & Horta-Baas, G. (2023). Gut-joint axis: Gut dysbiosis can contribute to the onset of rheumatoid

arthritis *via* multiple pathways. *Frontiers in cellular and infection microbiology, 13*, 1092118. https://doi.org/10.3389/fcimb.2023.1092118

Huang Z. Y., Stabler T., Pei F. X., Kraus V. B. (2016). Both Systemic and Local Lipopolysaccharide (LPS) Burden Are Associated With Knee OA Severity and Inflammation. *Osteoarthr. Cartil.* 24 (10), 1769–1775. doi: 10.1016/j.joca.2016.05.008
Wei, Z., Li, F., & Pi, G. (2022). Association Between Gut Microbiota and Osteoarthritis: A Review of Evidence for Potential Mechanisms and Therapeutics. *Frontiers in cellular and infection microbiology, 12*, 812596. https://doi.org/10.3389/fcimb.2022.812596
Boer C. G., Radjabzadeh D., Medina-Gomez C., Garmaeva S., Schiphof D., Arp P., et al.. (2019). Intestinal Microbiome Composition and Its Relation to Joint Pain and Inflammation. *Nat. Commun.* 10 (1), 4881. doi: 10.1038/s41467-019-12873-4

Yin, R., Zhang, K., Li, Y., Tang, Z., Zheng, R., Ma, Y., Chen, Z., Lei, N., Xiong, L., Guo, P., Li, G., & Xie, Y. (2023). Lipopolysaccharide-induced depression-like model in mice: meta-analysis and systematic evaluation. *Frontiers in immunology, 14*, 1181973. https://doi.org/10.3389/fimmu.2023.1181973

McDaniel, M., Jordan, I. A., Fox, S., & Younger, J. (2024). Investigation of Inflammation in Fibromyalgia After a Lipopolysaccharide-Induced Immune Response. *Journal of Pain*, 25(4), 34. https://doi.org/10.1016/j.jpain.2024.01.159

Jones C, Parkitny L, Strath L, Wagener BM, Barker A, Younger J. Altered response to Toll-like receptor 4 activation in fibromyalgia: A low-dose, human experimental endotoxemia pilot study. Brain Behav Immun Health. 2023 Nov 17;34:100707. doi: 10.1016/j.bbih.2023.100707. PMID: 38020479; PMCID: PMC10679487.

Benson, S., Engler, H., Wegner, A., Schedlowski, M., & Elsenbruch, S. (2020). Elucidating vulnerability to inflammation-induced hyperalgesia: Predictors of increased musculoskeletal pain sensitivity during experimental endotoxemia. *Brain Behavior and Immunity, 88*, 302–307. https://doi.org/10.1016/j.bbi.2020.06.022

Sabnis, A., Hagart, K. L., Klöckner, A., Becce, M., Evans, L. E., Furniss, R. C. D., Mavridou, D. A., Murphy, R., Stevens, M. M., Davies, J. C., Larrouy-Maumus, G. J., Clarke, T. B., & Edwards, A. M. (2021). Colistin kills bacteria by targeting lipopolysaccharide in the cytoplasmic membrane. *eLife, 10*, e65836. https://doi.org/10.7554/eLife.65836

Mondal, A. H., Khare, K., Saxena, P., Debnath, P., Mukhopadhyay, K., & Yadav, D. (2024). A Review on Colistin Resistance: An Antibiotic of Last Resort. *Microorganisms*, *12*(4), 772. https://doi.org/10.3390/microorganisms12040772

Daulatzai, M. A. (2015). Non-celiac gluten sensitivity triggers gut dysbiosis, neuroinflammation, gut-brain axis dysfunction, and vulnerability for dementia. *CNS & neurological disorders drug targets*, *14*(1), 110–131. https://doi.org/10.2174/1871527314666150202152436

Barbaro, M. R., Cremon, C., Stanghellini, V., & Barbara, G. (2018). Recent advances in understanding non-celiac gluten sensitivity. *F1000Research*, *7*, F1000 Faculty Rev-1631. https://doi.org/10.12688/f1000research.15849

Huang, Z., & Kraus, V. B. (2016). Does lipopolysaccharide-mediated inflammation have a role in OA?. *Nature reviews. Rheumatology*, *12*(2), 123–129. https://doi.org/10.1038/nrrheum.2015.158

Mendez, M. E., Sebastian, A., Murugesh, D. K., Hum, N. R., McCool, J. L., Hsia, A. W., Christiansen, B. A., & Loots, G. (2020). LPS-Induced Inflammation Prior to Injury Exacerbates the Development of Post-traumatic Osteoarthritis in Mice. *Journal of Bone and Mineral Research : the official journal of the American Society for Bone and Mineral Research*, *35*(11), 2229–2241. https://doi.org/10.1002/jbmr.4117

Hyperuricemia (High Uric Acid Level). (2024, May 1). Cleveland Clinic. https://my.clevelandclinic.org/health/diseases/17808-hyperuricemia-high-uric-acid-level

Shao, B., Lu, M., Katz, S. C., Varley, A. W., Hardwick, J., Rogers, T. E., Ojogun, N., Rockey, D. C., DeMatteo, R. P., & Munford, R. S. (2007). A Host Lipase Detoxifies Bacterial Lipopolysaccharides in the Liver and Spleen. *Journal of Biological Chemistry*, *282*(18), 13726–13735. https://doi.org/10.1074/jbc.m609462200

Luo, Y., Wu, Q., Meng, R., Lian, F., Jiang, C., Hu, M., Wang, Y., & Ma, H. (2023). Serum Uric Acid Levels and Their Association with Renal Function Decline and Kidney Disease Progression in Middle-Aged and Elderly Populations: A Retrospective Cohort Study. *Journal of multidisciplinary healthcare*, *16*, 3357–3366. https://doi.org/10.2147/JMDH.S435537

Choi HK, Atkinson K, Karlson EW, Curhan G. Obesity, Weight Change, Hypertension, Diuretic Use, and Risk of Gout in Men: The Health Professionals Follow-up Study. *Arch Intern Med*. 2005;165(7):742–748. doi:10.1001/archinte.165.7.742

Loeser R. F. (2010). Age-related changes in the musculoskeletal system and the development of osteoarthritis. *Clinics in geriatric medicine*, 26(3), 371–386. https://doi.org/10.1016/j.cger.2010.03.002

Leaky Gut Syndrome. (2024, May 1). Cleveland Clinic. https://my.clevelandclinic.org/health/diseases/22724-leaky-gut-syndrome

Yamamoto, Y., Miyagawa, Y., Kitazawa, M., Tanaka, H., Kuroiwa, M., Hondo, N., Koyama, M., Nakamura, S., Tokumaru, S., Muranaka, F., & Soejima, Y. (2020). Impact of barometric pressure on adhesive small bowel obstruction: a retrospective study. *BMC surgery*, 20(1), 168. https://doi.org/10.1186/s12893-020-00829-1

Chapter 10: When Good Food Is Bad for You
TheIHMC. (2014, November 24). Alessio Fasano, M.D.: *The gut is not like Las Vegas* [Video]. YouTube. https://www.youtube.com/watch?v=wha30RSxE6w

Bibbò, S., Pes, G. M., Usai-Satta, P., Salis, R., Soro, S., Quarta Colosso, B. M., & Dore, M. P. (2017). Chronic autoimmune disorders are increased in coeliac disease: A case-control study. *Medicine*, 96(47), e8562. https://doi.org/10.1097/MD.0000000000008562

He, M., Sun, J., Jiang, Z. Q., & Yang, Y. X. (2017). Effects of cow's milk beta-casein variants on symptoms of milk intolerance in Chinese adults: a multicentre, randomised controlled study. *Nutrition Journal*, 16(1). https://doi.org/10.1186/s12937-017-0275-0 Ref list Ursell, L. K., Metcalf, J. L., Parfrey, L. W., & Knight, R. (2012). Defining the human microbiome. *Nutrition reviews*, 70 Suppl 1(Suppl 1), S38–S44. https://doi.org/10.1111/j.1753-4887.2012.00493.x

Coburn, J. A., Vande Voort, J. L., Lahr, B. D., Van Dyke, C. T., Kroning, C. M., Wu, T. T., Gandhi, M. J., & Murray, J. A. (2013). Human leukocyte antigen genetics and clinical features of self-treated patients on a gluten-free diet. *Journal of clinical gastroenterology*, 47(10), 828–833. https://doi.org/10.1097/MCG.0b013e31828f531c

https://www.nytimes.com/2022/09/13/well/eat/food-sensitivity-test.html. (2022, September 13). *Nytimes.com.* https://www.nytimes.com/2022/09/13/well/eat/food-sensitivity-test.htm

Food Intolerance Versus Food Allergy. (n.d.). https://www.aaaai.org/tools-for-the-public/conditions-library/allergies/food-intolerance

The myth of IgG food panel testing | AAAAI. (n.d.). https://www.aaaai.org/tools-for-the-public/conditions-library/allergies/igg-food-test

Food allergy vs. food intolerance: What's the difference? (2024, February 28). Mayo Clinic. https://www.mayoclinic.org/diseases-conditions/food-allergy/expert-answers/food-allergy/faq-20058538

British Journal of Gastroenterology. (n.d.). British Journal of Gastroenterology. https://britishjournalofgastroenterology.com/food-allergen-elimination-for-obesity

Alcat vs. IgG Testing. (n.d.). https://cellsciencesystems.com/education/news/alcat-vs-igg-testing/

Cell Science Systems Reports Newly Discovered Cause of Delayed Food Allergies (Sensitivities). (n.d.). https://cellsciencesystems.com/education/research/cell-science-systems-reports-newly-discovered-cause-of-delayed-food-allergies-sensitivities Garcia-Martinez, I., Weiss, T. R., Yousaf, M. N., Ali, A., & Mehal, W. Z. (2018). A leukocyte activation test identifies food items which induce release of DNA by innate immune peripheral blood leucocytes. *Nutrition & metabolism, 15,* 26. https://doi.org/10.1186/s12986-018-0260-4

Yale researchers report on study of the efficacy of the Alcat Test for patients with irritable bowel syndrome and the pathomechanisms of food sensitivity. (n.d.). https://cellsciencesystems.com/education/webinars/yale-researchers-report-on-study-of-the-efficacy-of-the-alcat-test-for-patients-with-irritable-bowel-syndrome-and-the-pathomechanisms-of-food-sensitivity/

Landmark research published on the treatment of IBS. (n.d.). https://cellsciencesystems.com/education/research/landmark-research-published-on-the-treatment-of-ibs
Di Stefano, M., Pesatori, E. V., Manfredi, G. F., De Amici, M., Grandi, G., Gabriele, A., Iozzi, D., & Di Fede, G. (2018). Non-Celiac Gluten Sensitivity in patients with

severe abdominal pain and bloating: The accuracy of ALCAT 5. Clinical nutrition ESPEN, 28, 127–131. https://doi.org/10.1016/j.clnesp.2018.08.017

Jones, A. N., & Hansen, K. E. (2009). Recognizing the musculoskeletal manifestations of vitamin D deficiency. *The Journal of musculoskeletal medicine*, 26(10), 389–396.

Barhum, L. (2023, December 21). *What happens when calcium levels are low?* https://www.medicalnewstoday.com/articles/321865#complications

Carr, A. C., & McCall, C. (2017). The role of vitamin C in the treatment of pain: new insights. *Journal of translational medicine*, 15(1), 77. https://doi.org/10.1186/s12967-017-1179-7

Omega-3 Fatty Acids for Your Health | Arthritis Foundation. (n.d.). https://www.arthritis.org/health-wellness/treatment/complementary-therapies/supplements-and-vitamins/omega-3-fatty-acids-for-health

Shmagel, A., Onizuka, N., Langsetmo, L., Vo, T., Foley, R., Ensrud, K., & Valen, P. (2018). Low magnesium intake is associated with increased knee pain in subjects with radiographic knee osteoarthritis: data from the Osteoarthritis Initiative. *Osteoarthritis and cartilage*, 26(5), 651–658. https://doi.org/10.1016/j.joca.2018.02.002

Soppi E. T. (2018). Iron deficiency without anemia—a clinical challenge. *Clinical case reports*, 6(6), 1082–1086. https://doi.org/10.1002/ccr3.1529

Chapter 11: How Hormones Cause Joint and Muscle Pain
Cahalan, S. (2012). Brain on fire: my month of madness. New York, Simon & Schuster
Romm, A. (2024, May 8). *Women's Top Thyroid Questions, Answered.* Aviva Romm, MD. https://avivaromm.com/thyroid-questions/

Szczuko, M., Syrenicz, A., Szymkowiak, K., Przybylska, A., Szczuko, U., Pobłocki, J., & Kulpa, D. (2022). Doubtful Justification of the Gluten-Free Diet in the Course of Hashimoto's Disease. *Nutrients*, 14(9), 1727. https://doi.org/10.3390/nu14091727

Wentz, I. (2024, February 15). *Food Sensitivities and Hashimoto's—Dr. Izabella Wentz.* Dr. Izabella Wentz, PharmD. https://thyroidpharmacist.com/articles/food-sensitivities-and-hashimotos/

Rodolico, C., Bonanno, C., Pugliese, A., Nicocia, G., Benvenga, S., & Toscano, A. (2020). Endocrine myopathies: clinical and histopathological features of the major forms. *Acta myologica : myopathies and cardiomyopathies : official journal of the Mediterranean Society of Myology, 39*(3), 130–135. https://doi.org/10.36185/2532-1900-017

Moorman, P. G., Myers, E. R., Schildkraut, J. M., Iversen, E. S., Wang, F., & Warren, N. (2011). Effect of hysterectomy with ovarian preservation on ovarian function. *Obstetrics and gynecology, 118*(6), 1271–1279. https://doi.org/10.1097/AOG.0b013e318236fd12

Huang, Y., Wu, M., Wu, C., Zhu, Q., Wu, T., Zhu, X., Wu, M., & Wang, S. (2023). Effect of hysterectomy on ovarian function: a systematic review and meta-analysis. *Journal of ovarian research, 16*(1), 35. https://doi.org/10.1186/s13048-023-01117-1

Farland, L. V., Rice, M. S., Degnan, W. J., 3rd, Rexrode, K. M., Manson, J. E., Rimm, E. B., Rich-Edwards, J., Stewart, E. A., Cohen Rassier, S. L., Robinson, W. R., & Missmer, S. A. (2023). Hysterectomy With and Without Oophorectomy, Tubal Ligation, and Risk of Cardiovascular Disease in the Nurses' Health Study II. *Journal of women's health (2002), 32*(7), 747–756. https://doi.org/10.1089/jwh.2022.0207

Tinelli, A., Vinciguerra, M., Malvasi, A., Andjić, M., Babović, I., & Sparić, R. (2021). Uterine Fibroids and Diet. *International journal of environmental research and public health, 18*(3), 1066. https://doi.org/10.3390/ijerph18031066

Rouen, P. A., Krein, S. L., & Reame, N. E. (2015). Postmenopausal Symptoms in Female Veterans with Type 2 Diabetes: Glucose Control and Symptom Severity. *Journal of women's health (2002), 24*(6), 496–505. https://doi.org/10.1089/jwh.2014.4863

Lu, C. B., Liu, P. F., Zhou, Y. S., Meng, F. C., Qiao, T. Y., Yang, X. J., Li, X. Y., Xue, Q., Xu, H., Liu, Y., Han, Y., & Zhang, Y. (2020). Musculoskeletal Pain during the Menopausal Transition: A Systematic Review and Meta-Analysis. *Neural plasticity, 2020*, 8842110. https://doi.org/10.1155/2020/8842110

https://www.loyolamedicine.org/about-us/blog/menopause-related-musculoskeletal-pain

Fedotcheva, T. A., Fedotcheva, N. I., & Shimanovsky, N. L. (2022). Progesterone as an Anti-Inflammatory Drug and Immunomodulator: New Aspects in Hormonal

Regulation of the Inflammation. *Biomolecules, 12*(9), 1299. https://doi.org/10.3390/biom12091299

Cheng, L., & Wang, S. (2023). Lower serum testosterone is associated with increased likelihood of arthritis. *Scientific reports, 13*(1), 19241. https://doi.org/10.1038/s41598-023-46424-1

Parker, W. H., Broder, M. S., Liu, Z., Shoupe, D., Farquhar, C., & Berek, J. S. (2005). Ovarian conservation at the time of hysterectomy for benign disease. *Obstetrics and gynecology, 106*(2), 219–226. https://doi.org/10.1097/01.AOG.0000167394.38215.56

Rocca, W. A., Grossardt, B. R., de Andrade, M., Malkasian, G. D., & Melton, L. J., 3rd (2006). Survival patterns after oophorectomy in premenopausal women: a population-based cohort study. *The Lancet. Oncology, 7*(10), 821–828. https://doi.org/10.1016/S1470-2045(06)70869-5

December 25, 2006—Volume 28—Issue 24: Oncology Times. (n.d.). https://journals.lww.com/oncology-times/fulltext/2006/12250/study__prophylactic_oophorectomy_may_increase.

Frizziero, A., Vittadini, F., Gasparre, G., & Masiero, S. (2014). Impact of oestrogen deficiency and aging on tendon: concise review. *Muscles, ligaments and tendons journal, 4*(3), 324–328.

Wrzosek, M., Woźniak, J., & Włodarek, D. (2020). The causes of adverse changes of testosterone levels in men. *Expert review of endocrinology & metabolism, 15*(5), 355–362. https://doi.org/10.1080/17446651.2020.1813020

National Diabetes Statistics Report. (2024, May 15). Diabetes. https://www.cdc.gov/diabetes/php/data-research/index.html

Wei, G., Lu, K., Umar, M. et al. Risk of metabolic abnormalities in osteoarthritis: a new perspective to understand its pathological mechanisms. *Bone Res* 11, 63 (2023). https://doi.org/10.1038/s41413-023-00301-9

Libretexts. (2021, March 6). *13.27: Hormone Regulation.* Biology LibreTexts. https://bio.libretexts.org/Bookshelves/Introductory_and_General_Biology/Introductory_Biology_(CK-12)/13%3A_Human_Biology/13.27%3A_Hormone_Regulation

Suetomi, T., Ichioka, D., Iimura, T., Kojo, K., Ikeda, A., Kimura, T., Kawahara, T., Hoshi, A., Kandori, S., Negoro, H., & Nishiyama, H. (2022). 125 Characteristics of Testicular Atrophy During Testosterone Replacement Therapy (TRT). *The Journal of Sexual Medicine*, 19(Supplement_2), S175. https://doi.org/10.1016/j.jsxm.2022.03.398

McMahon, L. N., Handy, A. B., Jones, A. G., Mijares, S. A., Noon, A. E., & Meston, C. M. (2023). (100) The Effect of Oral Contraceptive Pill Type on Vulvovaginal Atrophy. *The Journal of Sexual Medicine*, 20(Supplement_2). https://doi.org/10.1093/jsxmed/qdad061.096

Monitoring HRT: Understanding the Evidence—DUTCH Test. (2024, April 3). DUTCH Test. https://dutchtest.com/video/monitoring-hrt-understanding-the-evidence/

Deprouw, C., Courties, A., Fini, J. B., Clerget-Froidevaux, M. S., Demeneix, B., Berenbaum, F., Sellam, J., & Louati, K. (2022). Pollutants: a candidate as a new risk factor for osteoarthritis-results from a systematic literature review. *RMD open*, 8(2), e001983. https://doi.org/10.1136/rmdopen-2021-001983

Sowers, M. et al (2006) Arthritis & Rheumatism Vol. 54, No. 8, Estradiol and Its Metabolites and Their Association With Knee Osteoarthritis, pp 2481–2487 DOI 10.1002/art.22005

Araújo, J., Cai, J., & Stevens, J. (2019). Prevalence of Optimal Metabolic Health in American Adults: National Health and Nutrition Examination Survey 2009-2016. *Metabolic syndrome and related disorders*, 17(1), 46–52. https://doi.org/10.1089/met.2018.0105

Dickson, B.M., Roelofs, A.J., Rochford, J.J. et al. The burden of metabolic syndrome on osteoarthritic joints. *Arthritis Res Ther* 21, 289 (2019). https://doi.org/10.1186/s13075-019-2081-x

Kohn, T. P., Louis, M. R., Pickett, S. M., Lindgren, M. C., Kohn, J. R., Pastuszak, A. W., & Lipshultz, L. I. (2017). Age and duration of testosterone therapy predict time to return of sperm count after human chorionic gonadotropin therapy. *Fertility and sterility*, 107(2), 351–357.e1. https://doi.org/10.1016/j.fertnstert.2016.10.004

Girum, T., & Wasie, A. (2018). Return of fertility after discontinuation of contraception: a systematic review and meta-analysis. *Contraception and reproductive medicine*, 3, 9. https://doi.org/10.1186/s40834-018-0064-y

Chapter 12:
Strittmatter M, Bianchi O, Ostertag D, Grauer M, Paulus C, Fischer C, et al. Altered function of the hypothalamic-pituitary-adrenal axis in patients with acute, chronic and episodic pain. *Schmerz*. 2005;19:109–16.

Carlesso, L. C., Sturgeon, J. A., & Zautra, A. J. (2016). Exploring the relationship between disease-related pain and cortisol levels in women with osteoarthritis. *Osteoarthritis and cartilage*, 24(12), 2048–2054. https://doi.org/10.1016/j.joca.2016.06.018
Chan, S., & Debono, M. (2010). Replication of cortisol circadian rhythm: new advances in hydrocortisone replacement therapy. *Therapeutic advances in endocrinology and metabolism*, 1(3), 129–138. https://doi.org/10.1177/2042018810380214

Fede, C., Petrelli, L., Guidolin, D., Porzionato, A., Pirri, C., Fan, C., De Caro, R., & Stecco, C. (2021). Evidence of a new hidden neural network into deep fasciae. *Scientific Reports*, 11(1). https://doi.org/10.1038/s41598-021-92194-z

Mediation for arthritis. (n.d.). Arthritis Society. https://arthritis.ca/treatment/pain-management/complementary-therapies/types-of-complementary-therapies/meditation-for-arthritis

Rodolico, C., Bonanno, C., Pugliese, A., Nicocia, G., Benvenga, S., & Toscano, A. (2020). Endocrine myopathies: clinical and histopathological features of the major forms. *Acta myologica : myopathies and cardiomyopathies : official journal of the Mediterranean Society of Myology*, 39(3), 130–135. https://doi.org/10.36185/2532-1900-017

Choi, J. C., Park, Y., Park, S. K., Lee, J. S., Kim, J., Choi, J. I., Yoon, K. B., Lee, S., Lim, D. E., Choi, J. Y., Kim, M. H., Park, G., Choi, S. S., & Lee, J. (2017). Testosterone effects on pain and brain activation patterns. *Acta Anaesthesiologica Scandinavica*, 61(6), 668–675. https://doi.org/10.1111/aas.12908

Daniyal M, Javaid SF, Hassan A, Khan MAB. The Relationship between Cellphone Usage on the Physical and Mental Wellbeing of University Students: A Cross-Sectional

Study. Int J Environ Res Public Health. 2022 Jul 30;19(15):9352. doi: 10.3390/ijerph19159352. PMID: 35954709; PMCID: PMC9368281.

Coskun A, Zarepour A, Zarrabi A. Physiological Rhythms and Biological Variation of Biomolecules: The Road to Personalized Laboratory Medicine. *International Journal of Molecular Sciences*. 2023; 24(7):6275. https://doi.org/10.3390/ijms24076275

Putting your phone down may help you live longer. (2024, April 19). *NYTimes.com*. https://www.nytimes.com/2019/04/24/well/mind/putting-down-your-phone-may-help-you-live-longer.html

Witters, B. D. (2024, February 7). U.S. Depression Rates Reach New Highs. *Gallup.com*. https://news.gallup.com/poll/505745/depression-rates-reach-new-highs.aspx Tabb, M., Gawrylewski, A., & DelViscio, J. (2024, February 20). Decoded: What Are Neurons? *Scientific American*. https://www.scientificamerican.com/video/decoded-what-are-neurons/

The Brain-Gut Connection. (2024, January 24). Johns Hopkins Medicine. https://www.hopkinsmedicine.org/health/wellness-and-prevention/the-brain-gut-connection Bendis PC, Zimmerman S, Onisiforou A, Zanos P, Georgiou P. The impact of estradiol on serotonin, glutamate, and dopamine systems. Front Neurosci. 2024 Mar 22;18:1348551. doi: 10.3389/fnins.2024.1348551. PMID: 38586193; PMCID: PMC10998471.

Appleton J. The Gut-Brain Axis: Influence of Microbiota on Mood and Mental Health. Integr Med (Encinitas). 2018 Aug;17(4):28-32. PMID: 31043907; PMCID: PMC6469458.

Gonzales GF, Carrillo C. Blood serotonin levels in postmenopausal women: effects of age and serum oestradiol levels. Maturitas. 1993 Jul;17(1):23-9. doi: 10.1016/0378-5122(93)90120-7. PMID: 8412840.

Paredes S, Cantillo S, Candido KD, Knezevic NN. An Association of Serotonin with Pain Disorders and Its Modulation by Estrogens. Int J Mol Sci. 2019 Nov 15;20(22):5729. doi: 10.3390/ijms20225729. PMID: 31731606; PMCID: PMC6888666.

Hannibal KE, Bishop MD. Chronic stress, cortisol dysfunction, and pain: a psychoneuroendocrine rationale for stress management in pain rehabilitation. Phys Ther. 2014 Dec;94(12):1816-25. doi: 10.2522/ptj.20130597. Epub 2014 Jul 17. PMID: 25035267; PMCID: PMC4263906.

Lee BH, Hille B, Koh DS. Serotonin modulates melatonin synthesis as an autocrine neurotransmitter in the pineal gland. Proc Natl Acad Sci U S A. 2021 Oct 26;118(43):e2113852118. doi: 10.1073/pnas.2113852118. PMID: 34675083; PMCID: PMC8639368.

Haack M, Simpson N, Sethna N, Kaur S, Mullington J. Sleep deficiency and chronic pain: potential underlying mechanisms and clinical implications. Neuropsychopharmacology. 2020 Jan;45(1):205-216. doi: 10.1038/s41386-019-0439-z. Epub 2019 Jun 17. PMID: 31207606; PMCID: PMC6879497.

Chapter 13: The Brain and Your Pain
Musculoskeletal Health Australia. (2018, December 5). *Pain, the brain and your amazing protectometer—Lorimer Moseley* [Video]. YouTube. https://www.youtube.com/watch?v=lCF1_Fs00nM

Chimenti RL, Post AA, Rio EK, Moseley GL, Dao M, Mosby H, Hall M, de Cesar Netto C, Wilken JM, Danielson J, Bayman EO, Sluka KA. The effects of pain science education plus exercise on pain and function in chronic Achilles tendinopathy: a blinded, placebo-controlled, explanatory, randomized trial. Pain. 2023 Jan 1;164(1):e47-e65. doi: 10.1097/j.pain.0000000000002720. Epub 2022 Jun 17. PMID: 36095045; PMCID: PMC10016230.

Booth J, Moseley GL, Schiltenwolf M, Cashin A, Davies M, Hübscher M. Exercise for chronic musculoskeletal pain: A biopsychosocial approach. Musculoskeletal Care. 2017 Dec;15(4):413-421. doi: 10.1002/msc.1191. Epub 2017 Mar 30. PMID: 28371175. Keysers C, Gazzola V. Hebbian learning and predictive mirror neurons for actions, sensations and emotions. Philos Trans R Soc Lond B Biol Sci. 2014 Apr 28;369(1644):20130175. doi: 10.1098/rstb.2013.0175. PMID: 24778372; PMCID: PMC4006178.

Nijs J, George SZ, Clauw DJ, Fernández-de-Las-Peñas C, Kosek E, Ickmans K, Fernández-Carnero J, Polli A, Kapreli E, Huysmans E, Cuesta-Vargas AI, Mani R, Lundberg M, Leysen L, Rice D, Sterling M, Curatolo M. Central sensitisation in chronic pain conditions: latest discoveries and their potential for precision medicine. Lancet Rheumatol. 2021 May;3(5):e383-e392. doi: 10.1016/S2665-9913(21)00032-1. Epub 2021 Mar 30. PMID: 38279393.

Karlsruher Institut für Technologie (KIT). (2017, October 25). Navigation system of brain cells decoded. *ScienceDaily*. Retrieved August 5, 2024, from www.sciencedaily.com/releases/2017/10/171025105041.htm

Traumatic Brain Injury. (n.d.). Johns Hopkins Medicine. https://www.hopkinsmedicine.org/health/conditions-and-diseases/traumatic-brain-injury

O'Keeffe M, O'Sullivan P, Purtill H, Bargary N, O'Sullivan K. Cognitive functional therapy compared with a group-based exercise and education intervention for chronic low back pain: a multicentre randomised controlled trial (RCT). Br J Sports Med. 2020 Jul;54(13):782-789. doi: 10.1136/bjsports-2019-100780. Epub 2019 Oct 19. PMID: 31630089; PMCID: PMC7361017.

Lin, H. M., Hsieh, P. S., Chen, N. C., Tsai, C. H., Kuo, W. F., Lee, Y. L., & Hung, K. C. (2023). Impact of cognitive behavior therapy on osteoarthritis-associated pain, insomnia, depression, fatigue, and physical function in patients with knee/hip osteoarthritis: A systematic review and meta-analysis of randomized controlled trials. *Frontiers in medicine*, 9, 1083095. https://doi.org/10.3389/fmed.2022.1083095

Erlenwein J, Diers M, Ernst J, Schulz F, Petzke F. Clinical updates on phantom limb pain. Pain Rep. 2021 Jan 15;6(1):e888. doi: 10.1097/PR9.0000000000000888. PMID: 33490849; PMCID: PMC7813551.

Subedi B, Grossberg GT. Phantom limb pain: mechanisms and treatment approaches. Pain Res Treat. 2011;2011:864605. doi: 10.1155/2011/864605. Epub 2011 Aug 14. PMID: 22110933; PMCID: PMC3198614.

Diaphragmatic Breathing. (n.d.). https://www.hopkinsmedicine.org/all-childrens-hospital/services/anesthesiology/pain-management/complimentary-pain-therapies/diaphragmatic-breathing#

Cherkin DC, Sherman KJ, Balderson BH, Cook AJ, Anderson ML, Hawkes RJ, Hansen KE, Turner JA. Effect of Mindfulness-Based Stress Reduction vs Cognitive

Behavioral Therapy or Usual Care on Back Pain and Functional Limitations in Adults With Chronic Low Back Pain: A Randomized Clinical Trial. JAMA. 2016 Mar 22-29;315(12):1240-9. doi: 10.1001/jama.2016.2323. PMID: 27002445; PMCID: PMC4914381.

Simic K, Savic B, Knezevic NN. Pain Catastrophizing: How Far Have We Come. Neurol Int. 2024 Apr 26;16(3):483-501. doi: 10.3390/neurolint16030036. PMID: 38804476; PMCID: PMC11130925.

Kent P, Haines T, O'Sullivan P, Smith A, Campbell A, Schutze R, Attwell S, Caneiro JP, Laird R, O'Sullivan K, McGregor A, Hartvigsen J, Lee DA, Vickery A, Hancock M; RESTORE trial team. Cognitive functional therapy with or without movement sensor biofeedback versus usual care for chronic, disabling low back pain (RESTORE): a randomised, controlled, three-arm, parallel group, phase 3, clinical trial. Lancet. 2023 Jun 3;401(10391):1866-1877. doi: 10.1016/S0140-6736(23)00441-5. Epub 2023 May 2. Erratum in: Lancet. 2023 Jun 17;401(10393):2040. doi: 10.1016/S0140-6736(23)01184-4. Erratum in: Lancet. 2023 Sep 16;402(10406):964. doi: 10.1016/S0140-6736(23)01905-0. PMID: 37146623.

Brain Facts—Healthy Brains by Cleveland Clinic. (2020, May 11). Healthy Brains by Cleveland Clinic. https://healthybrains.org/brain-facts/

Palmer KL, Shivgulam ME, Champod AS, Wilson BC, O'Brien MW, Bray NW. Exercise training augments brain function and reduces pain perception in adults with chronic pain: A systematic review of intervention studies. Neurobiol Pain. 2023 Apr 20;13:100129. doi: 10.1016/j.ynpai.2023.100129. PMID: 37206154; PMCID: PMC10189552.

Klyne, D. M., Barbe, M. F., James, G., & Hodges, P. W. (2021). Does the Interaction between Local and Systemic Inflammation Provide a Link from Psychology and Lifestyle to Tissue Health in Musculoskeletal Conditions? *International Journal of Molecular Sciences*, 22(14), 7299. https://doi.org/10.3390/ijms22147299

Lin, H. M., Hsieh, P. S., Chen, N. C., Tsai, C. H., Kuo, W. F., Lee, Y. L., & Hung, K. C. (2023). Impact of cognitive behavior therapy on osteoarthritis-associated pain, insomnia, depression, fatigue, and physical function in patients with knee/hip osteoarthritis: A systematic review and meta-analysis of randomized controlled trials. *Frontiers in medicine*, 9, 1083095. https://doi.org/10.3389/fmed.2022.1083095

Slimani, M., Tod, D., Chaabene, H., Miarka, B., & Chamari, K. (2016). Effects of Mental Imagery on Muscular Strength in Healthy and Patient Participants: A Systematic Review. *Journal of sports science & medicine, 15*(3), 434–450.

Borisovskaya, A., Chmelik, E., & Karnik, A. (2020). Exercise and Chronic Pain. *Advances in Experimental Medicine and Biology, 1228,* 233–253. https://doi.org/10.1007/978-981-15-1792-1_16

About the Author

Stacey Roberts PT, RN, MSN, is the co-founder of New You Health and Wellness and Positive Image Publishing. She received her physical therapy degree from Marquette University in 1990 and completed a sports medicine fellowship through the University of North Carolina Chapel Hill. Stacey obtained her MBA from Quantic School of Business and Technology and went on for her Master of Nursing from Alverno College. She has served as co-principle investigator in IRB-approved research related to shockwave and women's health. She has mentored over one hundred practitioners in Australia in the field of hormone optimization. Stacey was an adjunct professor for the Doctor of Physical Therapy program in the kinesiology department at University of Wisconsin, Milwaukee. She is the host of *The Pain Free Formula Podcast* and has authored three other books on women's health. Her clinic, New You Health and Wellness in Wauwatosa, Wisconsin, specializes in helping patients with muscle and joint pain, pelvic health and sexual health, as well as healthy fat loss and fitness, with a special focus on optimizing hormone and gut health.

Stacey Roberts PT, RN, MSN
New You Health and Wellness
10919 W Bluemound Rd, Suite 200
Wauwatosa, WI 53213

To receive a FREE discovery call, go to
www.newyouhealthandwellness.com
Email: info@newyouhealthandwellness.com
Call: 414 299 8121

Want to dig a little deeper?
Go to https://newyouhealthandwellness.com/ebooks to find out more about how to get rid of muscle and joint pain. And join us on The Pain Free Podcast at https://www.newyouhealthandwellness.com/the-pain-free-formula-podcast

www.ingramcontent.com/pod-product-compliance
Lightning Source LLC
Chambersburg PA
CBHW051523020426
42333CB00016B/1760